THE
OMEGA-3
EFFECT

Sears Parenting Library

The Baby Book
The Pregnancy Book
The Birth Book
The Premature Baby Book
The Portable Pediatrician
The Attachment Parenting Book
The Breastfeeding Book
The Fussy Baby Book
The Baby Sleep Book
The Vaccine Book
The Autism Book
The Discipline Book
The Healthiest Kid in the Neighborhood
The Family Nutrition Book
The A.D.D. Book
The Successful Child

Parenting.com FAQ Books

The First Three Months
How to Get Your Baby to Sleep
Keeping Your Baby Healthy
Feeding the Picky Eater

Sears Children's Library

Baby on the Way
What Baby Needs
Eat Healthy, Feel Great
You Can Go to the Potty

THE
OMEGA-3
EFFECT

• • •

EVERYTHING YOU NEED TO KNOW ABOUT
the **SUPERNUTRIENT** *for* **LIVING LONGER,**
HAPPIER, *and* **HEALTHIER**

WILLIAM SEARS, MD, WITH
JAMES SEARS, MD

Little, Brown and Company
New York Boston London

Little, Brown and Company
Hachette Book Group
237 Park Avenue, New York, NY 10017
littlebrown.com

First Edition: August 2012

Little, Brown and Company is a division of Hachette Book Group, Inc.,
and is celebrating its 175th anniversary in 2012.
The Little, Brown name and logo are trademarks
of Hachette Book Group, Inc.

Drawings by Deborah Maze

The publisher is not responsible for websites (or their content)
that are not owned by the publisher.

The Hachette Speakers Bureau provides a wide range of authors for
speaking events. To find out more, go to
hachettespeakersbureau.com or call (866) 376-6591.

ISBN 978-0-316-19684-0
Library of Congress Control Number 2012942129

10 9 8 7 6 5 4 3 2 1

RRD-C

Printed in the United States of America

Contents

• • •

Foreword

• • •

The book you are holding has been written by a doctor who shares with you his joy in good health and his love for his family and patients. Dr. Bill Sears wrote this book to "reach the *most* readers with the *best* science in the *simplest* way." During the past year, I saw him tirelessly work to develop stories and lessons that would help people understand how they might prevent and reverse habits that cause untold damage to their health and the health of their families.

As an experienced author, Dr. Bill knows to "keep it simple, make it fun" for his readers. As an experienced physician who has seen the tragic results of bad health habits and guidance, he knows that he must "keep it scientific, make it factual," he must avoid telling entertaining but misleading fantasies. You will enjoy seeing how he succeeds in giving science-made-simple explanations.

Although we have vast biomedical knowledge about disease, more than 80 percent of U.S. health care dollars are spent on issues caused by preventable lifestyle behaviors. Something is missing. *The Omega-3 Effect* makes us aware of what we need to understand and do to prevent this problem.

I happened to be a professor of biochemistry in 1964 when an article first reported that our bodies convert vitaminlike omega-3 and omega-6 fats into a complex set of powerful hormones. The next several decades were years of exciting discoveries, as hundreds of scientists uncovered even more important news about omega-3 and omega-6 hormones, including that they act on selective receptors located on nearly every cell and tissue of the body. As a result, these hormones affect nearly every physiological and pathological aspect of our lives. They play a role in many conditions, including atherosclerosis, thrombosis, arrhythmia, heart attacks, immune-inflammatory disorders, asthma, arthritis, psychiatric disorders, depression, suicide, oppositional behavior, unproductive workplace behaviors, cancer proliferation, and length of stay in hospitals.

The scope of the omegas' effects on our health is amazing. Although it has become common biomedical knowledge that omega-3 and omega-6 hormones are powerful enough to help prevent and treat many health problems, the incidence and prevalence of preventable diseases has not diminished. Enter Dr. Bill, who, like a patient Zen scholar, searched for simple metaphors that would shock the mind into awareness and lead readers to experience an enlightened or awakened state. He creates fresh views of how omega-3 nutrients help your heart, build smarter brains and better moods, help childhood learning and behavior, make pregnancies healthier and baby brains brighter, help balance inflammation, aid weight loss, keep you young, help you heal, and more. He helps you understand how the interaction between omega-3 and omega-6 fats is a key to good health. *The Omega-3 Effect* will make you aware of, and alive to, what you can do for your family and friends.

Bill Lands, PhD
Author of *Fish, Omega-3 and Human Health*
Fellow AAAS, ASN, SFRBM

Meet the Experts

• • •

A big helping of thanks to my board of advisers, who collectively have authored more than fifteen hundred scientific articles on health issues:

Tom Brenna, PhD. President of the International Society for the Study of Fatty Acids and Lipids (ISSFAL) in 2012; professor of human nutrition and chemical biology, Cornell University. His research mostly deals with studies on fatty acids and brain health.

Jørn Dyerberg, MD. One of the world's leading authorities on the health benefits of omega-3 fish oils. In the early 1970s he led a research team that studied the association between fish oil and heart disease in the Inuit population of Greenland.

William Harris, PhD. Omega-3 index coinventor; American Heart Association author; research professor, Sanford School of Medicine, University of South Dakota; senior scientist, Health Diagnostics Laboratory, Richmond, Virginia; president, Omega-Quant LLC.

Bruce Holub, PhD. Professor emeritus, Department of Human Health and Nutritional Sciences, University of Guelph, Ontario, Canada. Scientific director, DHA/EPA Omega-3 Institute, www .dhaomega3.org.

Penny Kris-Etherton, PhD. Distinguished professor of nutrition, Department of Nutritional Sciences, Pennsylvania State University. Her research includes over twenty years of clinical studies evaluating the role of diet on risk factors for cardiovascular disease.

Bill Lands, PhD. Author of *Fish, Omega-3 and Human Health*, second edition (AOCS Books, 2005). His website www .FastLearner.org discusses the omega balance scores of many foods. Professor Lands is credited with discovering the benefits of balancing the effects of excess omega-6 fatty acids with dietary omega-3 fatty acids, and he is widely regarded as one of the pioneering omega-3 researchers.

While I have for the most part followed the advice of these experts, occasionally even scientists differ in their interpretations of research studies, so some of my conclusions may not reflect the views of all my advisers.

THE
OMEGA-3
EFFECT

MY OMEGA-3 DISCLAIMER

Even though omega-3 EPA/DHA is the most thoroughly researched nutrient—discussed in some twenty-two thousand scientific articles—it is not a magical cure-all. Omega-3s in foods and supplements should not be considered a replacement for medicines prescribed by your doctor. Because you may have special medical needs, always consult your doctor about the right daily dosage of omega-3s for you, especially if you are taking prescription medications.

Go fishing online. The scientific and medical information about omega-3 EPA/DHA is continually changing. New therapeutic uses and dosages, recommended fish oil supplements, and safe-seafood updates are available at www.AskDrSears.com.

A SPECIAL THANKS

Thank you to Ocean Nutrition, Canada, for providing some financial and material support for this book, especially their underwriting of the 2011 Omega-3 Scientific Roundtable meeting.

Introduction

• • •

Fishing for the Omega-3 Effect

This book is about my twenty years of learning and living with the omega-3 effect. I hope that after reading it you will experience your own health benefits of omega-3s. I will take you on a journey through various cultures in the world and share with you stories that will change your life, as they have changed mine and the lives of many of my patients. In my medical practice, I have become more passionate about the health-promoting properties of omega-3 EPA/DHA than about any other nutrient. Having personally experienced the lifesaving qualities of this gift from the sea during my own health crisis and witnessed the omega-3 effect in my own patients, I feel compelled to share my "catch" with you. My wish for you is that after reading this book you will live a happier, healthier, and longer life.

Part I begins with the fish stories that gave rise to the idea for this book. I also take you fishing with some of the most trusted omega-3 scientists. Then, after you understand why I'm so passionate about omega-3s, you will get a science-made-simple explanation of the main omega fats you should know about, so that strange words like *eicosapentaenoic acid* (EPA) and *docosahexaenoic acid* (DHA) become familiar.

In Part II, I take you into my medical office for a series of visits addressing all your head-to-toe concerns. Imagine yourselves as patients coming to my office.

Part III features Dr. Bill's simple two-word prescription for nutritional health: "Go fish!" It includes a green-yellow-red traffic light list on how to select safe seafood. You will also learn how much seafood and fish oil supplements to take for the ailments you have.

After asking many patients in my medical practice what style of writing would best hold their attention, I selected the KISMIF principle: *keep it simple, make it fun.* I also wanted another KISMIF: *keep it scientific, make it factual,* to please the show-me-the-science readers. Any claim about a miracle nutrient releases the inner skeptic in them. They want authors to back up their statements with scientific references. So, in the notes section, I summarize some studies and cite many scientific references.

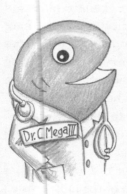

My China Story. Among my colleagues I'm known as the science-made-simple doctor. During my four speaking trips to China between 2009 and 2011, the chairperson of the Chinese Nutrition Society decided, "Put the American last on the program. He's funny and everyone will stay." My presentation opened, "Let me introduce my partner in medical practice, Dr. O. Mega III." Laughter was followed by a sip of green tea, which I took as a gesture of "like." Dr. O. Mega III was born one day in my office as I was explaining omega-3s to a patient, who then called me "the fish doctor." I imagined Dr. O. Mega III as a head-to-toe specialist, my partner in medical practice: a neurologist, ophthalmologist, pulmonologist, cardiologist, gastroenterologist, rheumatologist, dermatologist, and whatever other -ologist a patient would need.

THE EASIEST EXPLANATION OF WELLNESS AND ILLNESS

Wellness means keeping the sticky stuff from accumulating in your tissues; *illness* means too much sticky stuff accumulating in your tissues. Throughout this book you will learn how omega-3s tip you toward wellness.

My Roundtable Story. On April 27, 2011, after enjoying the traditional Sears salmon-at-sunset dinner the evening before, six of the top omega-3 researchers in the world gathered around our dining room table, including Dr. Jørn Dyerberg, the father of omega-3 research. In this first Omega-3 Effect Scientific Roundtable I was privileged to be surrounded by scientists who collectively had published more than fifteen hundred scientific articles. I had asked this panel of experts to help me critique the first draft of this book. My objective was to select the best science from the best scientists and translate it in a simple and entertaining way.

I opened the meeting by presenting the purpose of this book: "To reach the *most* readers with the *best* science in the *simplest* way." Lively discussions, constructive disagreements, and aha moments culminated in 106 pages of typed notes from the recorded session.

These experts scrutinized each page of the book to be sure the science was explained simply but accurately. Naturally, they allowed me a bit of poetic license when I challenged them to explain a complicated biochemical principle in simple and entertaining terms, such as, "Tom, imagine you're explaining this magical molecule to your mother." Occasionally, they couldn't get out of their white-coat laboratory lingo, and we laughed, saying, "See, that's why we need this book!" As we got deeper into the science in certain chapters, I realized that although there are thousands of published articles about the health benefits of omega-3 fats, there is solid science and soft science. These professionals knew the difference.

At the end of this memorable day I reminded my colleagues that one of the reasons their advice for this book was so brilliant and perceptive is that I had loaded them up with an omega-3 meal the evening before.

··· · · **PART I** · · · ··

WHAT YOU NEED TO KNOW ABOUT OMEGA-3S: SCIENCE MADE SIMPLE

After recounting four fish stories that prompted my interest in omega-3s, I take you inside the biochemistry of omega-3 fats to help you appreciate how this marvelous molecule is made and why it behaves so beautifully in your body and brain. I also clear up the standard consumer confusion about fats, explain why and how to give yourself an oil change, and point out that the key to good health is not necessarily a low-fat diet but rather a right-fat diet.

1

. . .

Four Fish Stories

The following stories tell about my search for a lifesaving nutrient and how discovering it enriched my health.

OUT OF THE MOUTHS OF BABES

My passion for omega-3 research began with the birth of our eighth child. The story begins in 1991 with the pregnant teenage daughter of a close friend. Like many pregnant teens, she was struggling with the realization that she did not have the maturity to raise her child. Yet, giving her child up for adoption was an even more upsetting alternative—choosing strange parents from a stack of résumés, perhaps never seeing her child again, and always wondering if she'd made the right decision.

Sensing her struggle, my wife, Martha, and I offered to raise her child in open adoption, where she could choose to be involved on her own terms. She was overjoyed, as were her parents, and she thrived throughout the rest of her pregnancy.

The Tale of Two Milks. Then came another decision that helped plant the seed for this book. Each of our previous seven children had been exclusively breast-fed. Although we wanted the same for the new baby—call her Lauren—we knew that Martha would only be able to produce half of what Lauren needed. Would Lauren be the first formula-fed Sears baby? No big deal, right? Wrong!

Around that time studies had started to show what breast-feeding mothers had suspected all along: children who are breast-fed grow up to be smarter and healthier.[1] We felt that just because Lauren was adopted, she shouldn't be deprived. We began searching for the formula closest to mother's milk.

After looking into the nutritional content of all the infant formulas, I discovered that every formula, especially those made in the United States, was missing vital brain-building omega-3 fats. The brain is 60 percent fat, and one of the top omega-3 fats in the brain is DHA. Hmm! Growing brains need special fats, yet infant formulas contained none. What's wrong with this cerebral picture? In the end, the only choice was to find a way to give Lauren breast milk. We concluded that the best alternative to her mother's milk was another mother's milk.

Two Mothers Making Milk. A few minutes after Lauren was born, she was nursing from her birth mom, who was producing colostrum, the perfect immune-boosting starter milk for a newborn. Meanwhile, Martha was hooked up to pumps trying to produce breast milk of her own. You should have seen the look on the obstetrical nurse's face when she came into the room and saw this dual-mom milk-making scene, probably the first and the last such scene of her career.

Milk Moms to the Rescue. The challenge was how to get enough breast milk for Lauren. During office visits mothers of infants would often comment on how much milk they were making. They were happy to give me the excess; at the end of each day I would leave the office with bottles of this liquid gold. Two years and thirty-five milk moms later, Lauren had made a smart nutritional start.

Improving the Formulas. What I learned from the failed formula search for our adopted baby made me angry. For more than ten years the known nutritional information about brain fats in human milk had been ignored by most formula makers, the Food and Drug Administration (FDA), and even my own profession. That had to change. I was motivated to "milk" the scientific literature for all the available facts. The more I read and studied about DHA in the brain, the more appalled I felt that millions of babies in much of the world went to bed each night without the most important brain-building fat. My crusade to get omega-3 smart fats into infant formulas began.

When I made my case to one of the largest formula sellers in the United States, I presented a slide show of what I thought was compelling proof for why omega-3 DHA, the smartest fat in the brain, must be added to infant formulas. To my amazement and disappointment, the head number cruncher said, "It would not be profitable for us to add DHA to our formula at this time because it would cost the consumer thirty-five cents more a can." Shocked, I pleaded, "I don't know a parent in the world who would not pay thirty-five cents more a day for their baby to grow a better brain!" I lost my case.

One of the joys of being a pediatrician is what I call the helper's high, the feeling that someone's life will be better because of something you said or did. Vowing to get formula companies to upgrade their offerings, I teamed up with doctors and scientists who taught me about brain-building fats, and continued crusading.

Finally, in 2001, the FDA and the infant formula companies could no longer ignore the science, and today nearly all companies add omega-3 fats to their infant formulas.

CANCER CAUSED ME TO CARE

Growing up Roman Catholic, I ate fish once a week. I thought I had to if I wanted to go to heaven. Yet what I ate were fish sticks and breaded fish sandwiches. Real seafood was not at the top of my list until April 1997, when I was diagnosed with colon cancer. Following major surgery, chemotherapy, and radiation therapy, I studied the data on survivors of major illnesses and life-changing events. Survivors had one thing in common: they made a project out of their problem. So that's what I did. Because my problem was in my gut, I began to search for the healthiest foods. Why not make a project out of healthy aging at the same time I was searching for the perfect health food? I found that the food that was ranked as the best health food also got top marks for healthy aging—seafood. In fact, the same fats that were crucial for baby brains were also important for senior brains and bodies. From head to toe—brain, eyes, heart, gut, muscles, joints, and skin—seafood was the best food to help prevent all the ailments I didn't want to get.

One of the earliest studies I discovered showed that cultures that eat more seafood have less cancer, especially colon cancer. In fact, these cultures have a lower incidence of just about every ailment of aging, like cardiovascular disease and many of the *-itis* illnesses, such as arth*itis*, bronch*itis*, and dermat*itis*. There was even emerging research suggesting these neuroprotective fats might delay Alzheimer's disease, or what I call cognitiv*itis*. In my life before cancer I was a hearty carnivore, habitually devouring grilled steaks. "Burn a big one" was my eating-out meat order. In my postcancer life I became a healthier kind of foodie, a seafood lover.[2]

INUITS DON'T GET HEART DISEASE

In order to learn more about omega-3 fats, I followed the advice I gave young medical students: "Surround yourself with wise mentors and have the wisdom and humility to learn from them."

In June 2006 I had the opportunity to spend a week fishing in Norway with a Danish doctor, Jørn Dyerberg, who is deservedly known as the father of omega-3s. After hearing of his thirty-plus years of research, I came home not only motivated to eat more fish with my family but also to share this research with my readers and patients.

As a medical resident in 1970, Dr. Dyerberg was intrigued by this paradox: Inuits ate a high-fat, high-cholesterol diet but enjoyed a low incidence of cardiovascular disease. That didn't fit with the conventional wisdom of the time, "Fat is bad for the heart." So Dr. Dyerberg traveled to Greenland to study the Inuits in the hope of finding a clue to this medical puzzle. While traveling through the Inuit villages he observed that the natives had frequent nosebleeds. Many people have nosebleeds in the winter. Must be the dry air in those igloos, he reasoned. Not so fast!

"Their nuisance nosebleeds seemed to take longer to stop than I remember occurring back home," he told me. When Dr. Dyerberg took blood samples from the Inuits, the tests revealed their bleeding times (the time it takes for blood to clot) were longer than the average bleeding times of Europeans. Could a high omega-fat diet cause thinner blood, he wondered? Many people on high-fat Western diets were dying of diseases related to blood that clotted too fast—at that time called the thick blood syndrome.[3]

Dr. Dyerberg continued to try to piece together the puzzle of longer bleeding times and lower incidence of heart disease. Could it be that when blood is slower to clot, arteries don't get plugged? Intrigued, he collected more blood samples from the

Inuits and then, back at home, compared them with similar blood samples from the Danes. Here's what he found:

Inuits' Advantages	Danes' Disadvantages
• Thinner blood, slower to clot	• Thicker blood, quicker to clot
• High blood level of omega-3 fats	• Low blood level of omega-3 fats
• Lower blood level of heart-unhealthy sticky fats	• Higher blood level of heart-unhealthy sticky fats
• Very low rates of cardiovascular disease	• High rates of cardiovascular disease
• A diet with much more omega-3 fat than omega-6 fat	• A diet with much more omega-6 fat than omega-3 fat
• Blood with balanced omega-3 and omega-6 fats	• Blood with too much omega-6 fat and too little omega-3 fat

Dr. Dyerberg realized that compared to the Danes, the Inuits ate more omega-3s (found in fish oils) and less of their cousins, the omega-6s (found in factory-processed foods).[4] Could there be a cause-and-effect relation here? Thirty years and over twenty thousand scientific articles later, the medical community had proved that one simple oil change could lower the rate of heart disease throughout the world.

Coincidentally, Dr. Dyerberg studied with Professor John Vane, who won the Nobel Prize for figuring out that aspirin worked by blocking the production of biochemicals that inflame the tissues. It's interesting that Dr. Dyerberg had a theory, later proven, that fish oil could have a similar therapeutic effect by a similar mechanism.

Dr. Dyerberg believed, and subsequent research confirmed, that the high doses of EPA in the Inuit diet lowered the risk of coronary artery thrombosis by shifting the tendency for blood's clotting too fast to clotting just right. When Inuits started eating like Americans, their blood began overclotting, and their rates of dying from cardiovascular disease became similar to the American rates. It's alarming that the relation between higher dietary proportions of omega-3s and lower incidence of heart disease was known in 1970, but as of 2012 the United States still does not have an official government Recommended Daily Intake (RDI) for omega-3s.

A year after our 2006 fishing trip and twice again in 2011, I had the pleasure of hosting Dr. Dyerberg at our home for the traditional Sears salmon-at-sunset dinner, where we caught up on the latest in omega-3 research and more fish stories. At one of our dinners I asked him to tell me more about his challenges in getting his discovery accepted by his medical colleagues.

When he studied blood platelets—those blood cells that bunch up and stick together—the Inuits' platelets contained a much higher proportion of omega-3s compared to the Danes', and their bleeding times were nearly twice as long. Dr. Dyerberg believed that the high proportion of omega-3 EPA fat in the Inuit diet shifted the blood to a slower-to-clot state and that the difference could help explain why the Inuits suffered fewer heart attacks.

Dr. Dyerberg went on to publish more than three hundred scientific articles on the health benefits of omega-3 fats. But these good fats had a public relations problem. The information about the good they do for bodies and brains lay hidden in journals that were not found in supermarkets. Finally, in the late 1990s, the popularity of omega-3 fats soared as top doctors began prescribing them as "medicine." All those -ologists started to use omega-3 EPA/DHA fats and saw that they were good. The cardiologists saw how much they helped hearts stay healthy. Ophthalmologists saw that they were good for the eyes. Neurologists saw how they built smarter brains. Gastroenterologists saw they were good for the gut. Rheumatologists found that they helped alleviate arthritis, and dermatologists discovered that omega-3 EPA/DHA

The Omega 3 Effect

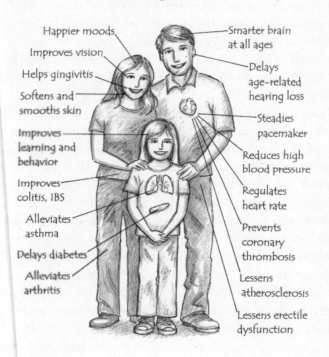

Happier moods

Improves vision

Helps gingivitis

Softens and smooths skin

Improves learning and behavior

Improves colitis, IBS

Alleviates asthma

Delays diabetes

Alleviates arthritis

Smarter brain at all ages

Delays age-related hearing loss

Steadies pacemaker

Reduces high blood pressure

Regulates heart rate

Prevents coronary thrombosis

Lessens atherosclerosis

Lessens erectile dysfunction

improved the skin. The list of medical problems alleviated by eating more omega-3 EPA/DHA is even longer.

MY MEDICINE MEAL

Much of this book was written under the influence of the omega-3 effect during my four lecture tours of Japan, the country with one of the highest per capita rates of seafood consumption and healthiest longevity. In Kyoto, Japan, in 2001 I was invited to speak about family health issues. Before the talk our host announced, "We will take you and Mrs. Sears out for a medicine meal." While I seldom eat a big lunch before giving a talk, it would have been rude to refuse. At the restaurant we were served a traditional meal, consisting of fifteen strange-looking small dishes, which our interpreter translated as "seafood and edible sea plants." Our host announced, "It's a Japanese tradition to feed visiting professors this medicine meal before their lecture. We find they give a better talk."

About an hour after my omega-3 overload, I felt the first effect — satisfied but not uncomfortably full. My lecture was in a hall adjacent to a famous Buddhist temple. After being escorted to the stage by the resident monk, I was amazed by the words that came out of my mouth. I experienced a level of alertness and eloquence that took me by surprise. Afterward Martha said, "That was your best talk yet." Those good gut feelings, together with a high cerebral alertness and mental peace, lasted several more hours. On three subsequent visits to Japan, I experienced similar omega-3 effects after prelecture medicine meals.

ENJOY THE OMEGA-3 EFFECT

Want your body to be in *biochemical balance?*
Want your brain to be *smarter?*
Want to feel *happier?*
Want your vision to be *sharper?*
Want your heart to be *stronger?*
Want your skin to feel *smoother?*
Want your pregnancy to be *healthier?*
Want your breast milk to be *more nourishing?*
Want your children to grow *smarter and healthier?*
Want your loved ones to live *longer?*

If you want any or all of these health perks, you want the omega-3 effect.

2

. . .

What Are Omega-3s and
Why Are They So Healthy?

This chapter explains what omega-3s are and why they are so good for you.

LET OMEGA-3S BE YOUR MEDICINE

Imagine you gather a group of people together to form a health club. In this club are people who already have ailments and want to reduce medication dependence. Also in the club are people who are well but don't want to wait until they get sick before they take care of themselves. They simply want to make their brains smarter and their bodies stronger, and to feel better and happier. Last, there are young parents or parents-to-be who plan ahead and want to give their children the best intellectual and physical start in life.

All of you decide to find the Top Doc in the world to give you the best science-based medicine to heal your hurts, prevent illnesses, and help your families thrive. I love that term *thrive*. It means being the healthiest you can be emotionally, intellectually, and physically.

You charter a plane and fly across the world to make an appointment with the Top Doc in preventive medicine. You enter the office and tell Top Doc why you're there and what you want. Top Doc hears your request and pleasantly surprises you: "I've got just the right medicine that all of you have come searching for."

You're all imagining what this marvelous medicine could be. To add to your surprise, you don't see Top Doc reaching for a prescription pad. Instead, she reaches into a drawer and hands you a fish. She reaches into another drawer and hands you a bottle of fish oil.

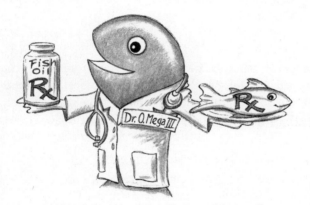

Top Doc's "prescriptions" receive mixed reactions. Most are amazed, some are confused, some even incredulous. Some wonder why they traveled all this way to get a fish and a bottle of fish oil.

To calm their anxiety, Top Doc says, "I sense your confusion. When you came here you gave me a list of your ailments and your wishes, and challenged me to help heal your hurts. Some of you have early Alzheimer's disease. Others suffer from poor vision. Many of you have arthritis or some other *-itis*. Many have cardiovascular disease. A few have diabetes. Many of you have mood disorders. And I see there are a few expectant and new moms here who simply want to raise smarter and healthier babies. You asked me for the most scientifically researched, safest medicine for all these needs, and that's what I'm giving you. My medicine is certainly not *instead of* the prescription drugs your own doctor recommends, but it also is very well researched."

Sensing the sincerity in this doctor's voice, the eager crowd upgrades their impressions from "something is fishy here" to "I'm glad we consulted this Top Doc!"

Sound farfetched? Here are quotes from some of the Top Docs whose advice I trust:

As a doctor, I believe omega-3s are one of the rare magic bullets in medicine.

—*Mehmet Oz, MD*[1]

Because of omega-3 deficiency in our troops they are at increased risk of physical and psychological illnesses. We want our troops to benefit from this new omega-3 science.

—*Surgeon General Richard Carmona,*
at a Nutrition for Warfighters Conference[2]

THE LANGUAGE OF LIPIDS MADE SIMPLE

Because more misinformation is circulated about fats (also called lipids) than about any other nutrient, here's a slim course on fat terms you should know. If your brain could vote, it would pick fats as the most important nutrient. The heart would second that.

Unsaturated Fats. On the fat molecules are empty areas; let's call them parking spaces. When there is plenty of room to park, these fats are called unsaturated. If lots of spaces are unfilled, the fat is called a highly unsaturated fatty acid (HUFA). HUFAs are the healthiest fats because they are liquid, smooth, soft, and flexible. In fact, because they are so flexible, they become liquid and are called oils, namely, the omega oils.

Biochemically speaking, these parking spaces are called double bonds. These double bonds are the usual areas that other chemicals attach to, either naturally or put there by food chemists. If oxygen attaches to these double bonds ("oxidize"), they spoil or turn rancid. Think of fish exposed to air. If they are zapped with hydrogen molecules (e.g., trans fats or hydrogenated oils), they get stiff but don't spoil. If they stay the way nature intended (neither oxidized nor hydrogenated), they remain healthfully soft, elastic, flexible, and adaptable.

Saturated Fats. Along come cars (hydrogen molecules) that fill some or all of the parking spaces. The more parking spots that are filled, the more saturated the parking lot fat molecule becomes. Because these parking spots are filled, the molecule becomes stiff. Like HUFAs, these saturated fats are healthy building blocks for tissues that require some stiffness, such as the myelin of the brain. As long as the HUFAs and saturated fats are eaten in the right proportions, the tissue is healthy.

Hydrogenated Fats. Along comes an unscrupulous builder who decides to change the normal configuration of the parking spaces from natural to unnatural (resulting in trans fats, meaning the molecule is chemically crossed up), and the parking spaces are zapped with hydrogen cars (hydrogenated fats). This chemical mischief makes the fat molecule so stiff and sticky that other cars (e.g., oxygen) won't park there. So the parking lot stays the same (hydrogenated fat sits on the shelf and doesn't spoil for years).

Tissues love HUFAs because they act like a multipurpose building material, changing shape to become whatever growing and healing tissue needs.

INTRODUCING OMEGA-3S

Let me introduce you to the omega-3 fish oil medicines. I use the term *medicine* to mean any chemical, food, herb, or spice that helps your body heal and be healthier. This could be a prescription pill or a nutrient in food. Remember, one of the most famous medical doctors, Hippocrates, called food "medicine." My favorite medicine is omega-3 fish oil. And the good health omega-3s give you I call the omega-3 effect. Omega-3s are the safest, most healing and health-producing medicines that I prescribe.

Omegas Are Flexible Fats. The best fats are smooth, soft, and flexible. The worst fats are stiff and sticky. Most illnesses are caused by an accumulation of stiff and sticky fats in your tissues, such as the brain and heart. Here is the simplest explanation of illness and wellness you've ever heard. I call it my sticky stuff cause of disease. You put stiff and sticky fats in your mouth, you get stiff and sticky stuff in your tissues (illness). You put smooth and flexible fats (omega-3s) in your mouth, you get smooth and soft tissues (wellness).

You can tell a lot about how fats will behave in your body by how they appear in food. Some fats are stiff, like lard and the marbling in steak. When you eat them, they behave the same way in your body, making your arteries stiff. Older folks (and even kids) get hardening of the arteries after years of eating stiff fats. What makes omega-3s so healthful is that these fats act as fluidly in your body as fish swim in the sea. Omega-3s keep your tissues soft and smooth.

A fat molecule is like a necklace. Each bead on the necklace is a carbon atom. There are also flexible areas on the molecule called double bonds, which bend like hinges. In general, the longer the necklace, and the more carbon atoms and hinges the molecule has, the more flexible and healthful is the effect of the fat in the body.

A necklace whose beads are held together by string is softer and more flexible than a necklace made of wire, which is stiffer and can't bend as well. Fat molecules whose hinges bend easily are called unsaturated. Fat molecules with stiff hinges are called saturated because hydrogen atoms fill up (saturate) the double bonds, making them stiffer. Some saturated fats have no hinges at all.

Omega-3 EPA/DHA ("the tall guys") have more carbon atoms (20–22 atoms) and more hinges (5–6 double bonds) than fats like ALA (the "short guys"), with 18 carbon atoms and 3 hinges.

Remember, health and wellness means having soft and smooth tissues. Illness is usually caused by stiff and sticky tissues. This is why, when doctors talk about the biochemical basis of disease, they say, "The tissue is the issue."[3]

In the body omega-3s are known as quick-change artists. They can change shape and quickly become whatever your tissue needs them to be for growth, function, and repair. The flexible hinges on omega-3 molecules help them assume all kinds of unusual shapes and wriggle into whatever part of the tissue needs more omega-3s.

KNOW YOUR OMEGAS

Omega-3s are so named because omega is the last letter of the Greek alphabet, and most of these fats' healthful qualities are at the tail end of the molecule. The 3 refers to a soft spot (double bond) like a hinge, on the third carbon atom from the end. This hinge makes the molecule soft and flexible.

More omegas will probably be discovered in the future, but the following ones are the most popular omegas that you should know about now.

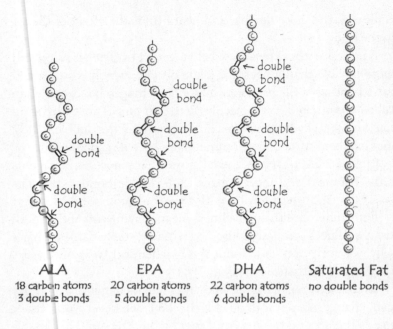

ALA	EPA	DHA	Saturated Fat
18 carbon atoms	20 carbon atoms	22 carbon atoms	no double bonds
3 double bonds	5 double bonds	6 double bonds	

ALA (Alpha Linolenic Acid)

Found in plants like salad greens and in seeds like flax and canola, ALA is the most abundant omega-3 fat in nature. It is a "short guy" in that it has only 18 carbon atoms and 3 hinges. Since, for tissue health, the body and brain prefer "tall guys" (like the omegas EPA and DHA), the body must use enzymes to convert ALA to EPA and DHA. Enzymes are the body's micromechanics that convert ALA into EPA and DHA, fashioning them into the tissue the body needs to grow and repair. Conversions like these are very inefficient. Only 1–4 percent of the omega-3 ALA oils you eat may be converted to EPA and even less to DHA. People vary in how well their individual biochemistry can convert ALA into EPA and DHA. (See more about ALA conversion in flax oil, page 164.)

EPA (Eicosapentaenoic Acid)

This "tall guy" omega-3 molecule, found mainly in seafood, has 20 carbon atoms and 5 double bonds. (Its name, of Greek origin, reflects this: *eicosa,* 20; *penta,* 5; *enoic,* refers to double bond.) Like other omega-3s, EPA has its first hinge third from the end of the molecule. It has more hinges and carbon atoms than ALA and is therefore more flexible.

DHA (Docosahexaenoic Acid)

Also found mainly in seafood, this "tall guy" omega-3 has 22 carbon atoms and 6 double bonds (*docosa,* 22; *hexa,* 6). Like EPA, it is a HUFA, or highly unsaturated fat.

Most of us need to eat more of these three amigos, ALA, EPA, and DHA.

Omega-6 Fats

The first double bond of omega-6 fats is on the sixth carbon atom from the end of the molecule. There are two kinds of omega-6s: linoleic acid (LA), found mainly in seeds and oils, and arachidonic acid (AA, sometimes abbreviated ARA), found mainly in meat and dairy products.

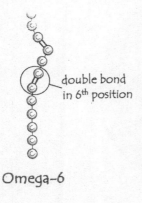

double bond in 6th position

Omega-6

Most people across the world have an insufficiency of omega-3 EPA and DHA but enough, or even an excess of, omega-6s. Therefore, most people need to eat more omega-3 fish oil but rarely need to eat more omega-6 oil.

Suppose you were an omega fatty acid applying for a job in any cell of the body. You approach the CIA, or Cellular Intelligence Agency: "Hi, I'm a HUFA, a *highly* *useful* *flexible* *agent.* I can do any job you need me to do. I protect and repair, and help you grow and heal. And I help translate your secret signals from one cell to another."

"Come right in. We need you," the cell says. "Each day we're attacked by sticky stuff that humans call food."

OMEGAS ARE MEMBRANE MOLECULES

Suppose you go to your doctor for treatment of various complaints. Your doctor takes a nutritional history, noting your omega-3 intake, and measures the level of omega-3s in your blood. Surprisingly, she says, "You suffer from the leaky cell membrane syndrome." You have no idea what that is, but leaky cell membranes don't sound good.

Cell membranes are like flexible bags that protect the energy-building and genetic material inside the cell. In fact, there is a medical truism: Your body is only as healthy as each cell in it. That makes sense because our bodies are composed of trillions of cells. Omega-3s

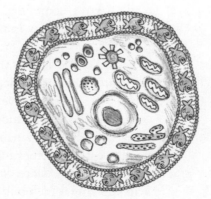

are called the membrane molecules because they make the cell membranes healthier. Cell membranes are selective, which makes them protective. They let good nutrients seep into the cell through the bloodstream while keeping the bad stuff, like toxins, out.

If you think about the marvelous structure of a cell membrane, and appreciate its design, you'll want to eat more omega-3s. Imagine a cell membrane. It is in contact with liquids on two sides: on the outside it touches blood and other body fluids. On the inside, it is in contact with fluid cell contents, which it must protect because the inside of each cell is the body's growth, repair, and energy network. A cell membrane needs to be selectively permeable, allowing good nutrients to seep through while keeping toxins out. Each cell membrane contains millions of miniature entry doors, called receptors, through which nutrients are transported into the cell for use and waste is sent back out into the bloodstream.

Healthy cell membranes are the perfect balance of stiff (saturated) fats and flexible (unsaturated) fats. If you suffer from an omega-3 dietary deficiency, your cell membranes are stiff and leaky. Omega-3s, the flexible fats, help fashion the fluidity of the cell membrane, enabling it to adjust to its ever-changing environment. Omega-3s also act like the membrane's maintenance engineers by producing chemical messengers, called prostaglandins, that protect the cell membrane from harm and enable it to transport the nutrients it needs.

To give an example, people with type-2 or insulin-resistant diabetes have stiff and leaky membranes. If the cell membrane is omega-3-deficient, the doors, or receptors, on the cell membrane are stiff and less receptive to insulin.

THE DIFFERENCES IN FATS

The flexible fats, the omegas, are also known as HUFAs (highly unsaturated fatty acids). Remember, HUFAs are healthy. Popular publications often write about "good fats," "bad fats," "low-fat diets," and so on. Those terms can be misleading.

To be clear, all fats naturally found in foods that come from the sea or flourish on the land are good fats. The fake fats made in factories (e.g., hydrogenated oils) are bad fats. And sometimes it's an *excess* of good fats (e.g., too much saturated or animal fat) that can be bad for you. Most people need to eat a *right-fat* diet rather than a low-fat diet.

Fishermen believe that the omega-3 fats in krill and other seafood that fish eat keep the muscles and blood vessels of fish flexible, even in freezing water, and that omega-3s seem to have the same effects on human tissues.

GIVE YOURSELF AN OIL CHANGE

An oil change is one of the healthiest and most needed dietary changes a person at any age can make. Making these oil changes can help you think smarter, feel better, and live longer.

Oil Change #1: Eat More Omega-3 Oil

This is the healthiest oil change you can make. Even if you just make this one oil change, you are likely to feel healthier from head to toe. Yet, to enjoy an even greater omega-3 effect, consider adding a second dietary oil change.

Oil Change #2: Eat Less Omega-6 Oil

In recent years a growing number of scientists and health educators have suggested that while eating more omega-3 oil is most important for optimal health, some people need one additional oil change: *eat less omega-6 oil*. They propose that *omega balance* should be the ultimate goal. New insights reveal that the imbalance of excess omega-6 and insufficient omega-3 in tissues may be the root cause of many chronic diseases, especially inflammation or -*itis* illnesses. (See Chapter 7 for more about inflammation.)

Oil Change #3: Eat Very Little Hydrogenated Oil

Besides eating more omega-3 oil, especially omega-3 EPA/DHA fish oil, eat less chemically modified oil like hydrogenated oil.

In addition, replace much of the animal-based saturated fat in your diet with the omega oils to prevent omega oil insufficiency. Do not replace saturated fats with junk carbohydrates. The low-fat diets and the consequent increase in junk carbs in the standard American diet (SAD) are among the most unhealthy changes in U.S. nutritrional history. In fact, new thinking among cardiovascular researchers is that saturated fats may not be associated with increased risk of cardiovascular disease as much as an increase in dietary junk carbs.

These are the oil changes that most nutritionists and omega-3 scientists agree upon and that science most supports.

UNDERSTANDING OMEGA BALANCE

Omega balance means eating sufficient omega-3 and omega-6 oils in the proper balance. You may read that the optimal ratio of omega-6s to omega-3s is about 3:1 (the ratio in the standard American diet is 10:1 or more). But the problem with ratios is that you could be deficient in both oils, especially omega-3s, yet still have the right ratio. Proponents of omega balance teach that we should not only eat more omega-3 fish oil but less omega-6 oil (such as corn, soy, and cottonseed oils, which make up as much as 20 percent of the standard American diet). However, I'm concerned that this theory leads consumers to believe that omega-6s are bad fats, which is not true. For example, nuts are real food with a high omega-6 to omega-3 ratio. To reject nuts simply because they have this high ratio and to compare them with factory-made foods, such as potato chips, with a similar high ratio is, shall we say, nuts! Omega-6s are good fats, essential to the health of every organ in the body and a partner to omega-3s in preventive medicine. As I've said before, fats that Mother Nature makes are good fats. It's their *excess* that causes them to have a bad effect in the body.

THE OMEGA-6 BULLY EFFECT

Tissues, especially cell membranes, need both omega-3s and omega-6s. These two omegas are like friends who play together and build together. When they play nicely and don't try to overpower each other, they build healthy tissues. But when there is an excess of omega-6, it tends to bully and overpower omega-3, especially ALA. Within the cell membranes are built-in biochemicals called enzymes. Like bricklayers, these enzymes assemble these two fats to build and maintain a structurally sound cell

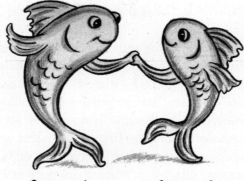

Omega-6   Omega-3

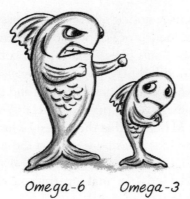

Omega-6   Omega-3

membrane. One of these enzymes is cleverly called *elongase*; it adds carbon atoms to the shorter molecule to make it longer (a "tall guy"). It converts ALA into EPA and DHA.

Many scientists believe that there are only so many tissue enzymes to go around.[4] When we eat too many omega-6s, commonly found in the standard American diet (SAD), they use up most of the enzymes, leaving too few to help the cells use the omega-3s and convert ALA into EPA/DHA. When tissues have an excess of omega-6s and a deficiency of omega-3s, the body will have an inflammatory imbalance, meaning that wear and tear takes over repair. The excess omega-6 effect dilutes the omega-3 effect. A very important point made at our Omega-3 Effect Scientific Roundtable: if you eat sufficient omega-3s, you will automatically decrease your tissue levels of excess omega-6s.

Other scientists believe that it's only EPA/DHA deficiency that's the problem, not omega-6 excess.[5] They conclude that if you just eat enough omega-3 EPA/DHA oil, you won't have to worry about eating less omega-6 oil. They support the idea that eating sufficient omega-3 EPA/DHA automatically lowers the level of omega-6 (especially arachidonic acid, the most proinflammatory omega-6 in the body) and that this is more important than simply eating less omega-6. These scientists say that the inflammatory effects of excess omega-6 won't occur if you simply eat more omega-3 EPA/DHA.

Omega-6 oils have gotten a bad rap because of the company they keep. Many food processors load up their chemical foods with cheap omega-6 oils like soy, corn, and cottonseed oils, the darlings of the food industry. True, Americans are eating more of these chemical foods and getting fatter and sicker, but is that because of the omega-6 oils per se or because they're put in so many junk foods? I believe that the omega-6s have become guilty by association. Besides advising you to eat more omega-3 oil and less omega-6 oil, I would say, eat more real foods and fewer factory-processed foods. In making this oil change, you will automatically eat less omega-6 oil.

In line with the theme of "the tissue is the issue," here's another reason I personally started eating more omega-3 oil and less omega-6 oil. When fish farmers grain-feed their fish a high omega-6 diet, the amount of omega-6 in the fish flesh goes way

Your Oil Change Guide

Best	Better[a]	Bad
Fish oil	Corn oil	Partially hydrogenated oils,
Flax oil	Soy oil	trans fats
Olive oil	Safflower oil[b]	Lard
	Sunflower oil[b]	
	Coconut oil[c]	
	Canola oil[d]	

a. These are not bad fats, as they are often portrayed; rather, the fake food they're put into is bad. Enjoy these oils in moderation.

b. The high oleic version is better because of the added effect of lowering sticky blood fats and it adds shelf life.

c. Coconut oil is making a comeback as a healthy oil. Best is *virgin* coconut oil.[6]

d. Because canola oil is high in omega-3 ALA (not EPA/DHA), some would put this healthy oil in the "best" category. See www.AskDrSears.com for up-to-date information on these oils.

up. So their tissues no longer enjoy an optimal omega balance. (See Chapter 12.) I don't want my tissues to get the proinflammatory effect of the high omega-6 diet as did the farmed fish that were fed fake food. So I eat like a wild fish: more omega-3 and less omega-6.

Based upon my detective work and on the advice of my omega-3 effect expert advisers, I conclude that in order to achieve omega balance, you should

- eat sufficient omega-3s: more oily seafood, adequate fish oil supplements, and/or omega-3 supplemented foods;
- eat more real foods and fewer processed foods.

OMEGA QUESTIONS YOU MAY HAVE

Omega-3s in Foods

Why don't food manufacturers simply add more omega-3 and less omega-6 to, say, potato chips?

As usual, the answer is money and taste. Fish oils are more expensive than plant oils, and they spoil faster. While it may seem unfair, the healthier the fat, the quicker it spoils. Although more hinges make for a healthier fat, that's a mixed blessing. Unlike the stiffer fats with fewer hinges (saturated fats like butter), flexible (unsaturated) fats are very fragile. This makes them susceptible to oxidation, or "rust," as when a cut avocado turns brown or fish smells "fishy" when exposed to air for a long time. So if you put omega-3s in processed foods and set them on the shelf, they could spoil. That's why fish have to be eaten soon after you catch or thaw them. However, by a new method, omega-3s *can* be added to foods without spoiling (see the next question).

No Fishy Taste

I've happily noticed that some foods, such as chips and chewies, with "omega-3 EPA/DHA added" have no fishy taste. Why?

A recent scientific breakthrough, called microencapsulation, wraps the omega-3 molecules in a biochemical capsule to make them more stable when added to foods. This protective wall locks in the health benefits of omega-3s while locking out any taste or smell. This keeps them fresh in the food for a long time so they don't spoil. With this new technology, omega-3s are stable and don't spoil quickly, so they are being added to an increasing number of popular foods.

Omega Balance for Babies

I'm pregnant. Should I eat less omega-6 oil besides eating more omega-3s?

Yes, babies need both. During the stages of most rapid brain growth—pregnancy to infancy—it is smart to eat more omega-3s and cut down on the usual *excess* of omega-6 oils.[7] A sufficient diet of both of these omegas is necessary for optimal brain growth. Remember, the primary goal at all ages, especially during infancy and pregnancy, is an omega-3 sufficiency. Most mothers eat enough omega-6 oils so they don't have to supplement with them. But most need to eat more omega-3s. And, I would add, for all ages, Eat more real foods and fewer factory foods.

Saturated Fats

I've read that eating too much saturated fat is bad for you. Why?

The three oil changes that nearly every expert agrees you should make:

* Eat more omega-3s, fish fats.
* Eat fewer saturated fats, such as meat fats.
* Eat as little as possible of fake oils, hydrogenated oils, or trans fats.

Historically, health articles are awash with fat-bashing pseudoscience. Sat-fat bashing began several decades ago when statistical studies showed that people who eat too much saturated fat, especially animal fat, have a higher incidence of heart disease. But healthy tissues need saturated fats as well as omega-6 oils. After all, saturated fats make up the bulk of some tissues like myelin, the white matter of the brain. It's eating *excess* saturated fats from animal products that may harm your heart. The American Heart Association recommends limiting saturated fats, especially those in meat, to no more than 7 percent of daily calories.

Some sat-fat put-downs were based more on marketing and money than on science. The corn and soy oil industry criticized healthy tropical oils as "high in saturated fat." Yet coconut oil is making a comeback in light of new science showing that it behaves in the body in a more tissue-friendly way (less sticky stuff in blood vessels) than the saturated fats in meats. Saturated fats are not bad fats. It's eating them in excess that can be bad for your health. That's why one of the themes of this book is *eat more fats from fish and fewer from meat.*

Omega-3-Deficient? How to Tell

How can I tell if I have an omega-3 deficiency?

Two clues that you are omega-3-sufficient: Do you eat at least 12 ounces of oily seafood weekly or take at least 1000 milligrams

YOUR OMEGA-3 EFFECT CHECKLIST

Omega-3s are a head-to-toe healing nutrient. Here's a list of the ailments that science suggests omega-3s can help heal and an omega-3 deficiency can make worse. Check each problem you or a loved one has.

- ❑ ADHD/ADD (attention deficit hyperactivity disorder) and learning disorders
- ❑ Age-related hearing loss
- ❑ Allergies
- ❑ Alzheimer's disease, dementia
- ❑ ARMD (age-related macular degeneration)
- ❑ Arthritis
- ❑ Asthma
- ❑ Autism
- ❑ Blood vessel thrombosis
- ❑ Bone density, weak
- ❑ Bronchitis
- ❑ Cancer
- ❑ Colitis
- ❑ Depression and anxiety
- ❑ Dermatitis
- ❑ Diabetes

- ❑ Dry eyes
- ❑ Eczema, psoriasis
- ❑ Gingivitis
- ❑ Hearing loss
- ❑ Heart arrhythmias
- ❑ Heart attack
- ❑ Heart failure
- ❑ High blood pressure
- ❑ Hot flashes
- ❑ Inflammatory bowel disease
- ❑ Menstrual pains
- ❑ Migraines
- ❑ Mood disorders, bipolar disorder
- ❑ Multiple sclerosis
- ❑ Obesity
- ❑ Rheumatoid arthritis
- ❑ Stroke
- ❑ Traumatic brain injury

(mg) of omega-3 fish oil supplements daily? If so, you are likely to be omega-3-sufficient. Also, you can get an omega-level blood test to give you a clue. (See blood test, page 160.) In addition, see the checklist I give patients in my medical practice. You may wonder why it is so long. Omega-3s help every cell in the body be healthier. If the cells are omega-3-deficient, it follows that the organs they make up are as well.

- All four omegas—ALA, EPA, DHA, and omega-6s—are necessary for optimal health.
- Eat sufficient omega-3s. (See dosages, Chapter 11.)
- If you have special nutritional situations, such as -*itis* illnesses, consider eating more EPA and DHA oils and less omega-6 oil.
- Eat more real foods, fewer processed factory foods.

THE HEAD-TO-TOE HEALING EFFECTS OF OMEGA-3S

Imagine that you are one of the growing number of people who realize that the answer to our health care crisis is self-care. You want to take charge of your health. To help you get started on your personal health plan, embark on a series of appointments with me, Dr. Bill, to learn how to heal the hurts you already have and to get preventive medicine advice to keep your body healthy. During your office visits you will meet Dr. Bill's imaginary partner in medical practice, Dr. O. Mega III, who dispenses her omega tips to remember.

Kids who eat more omega-3s see better and think better.
— *Cornell University neurology researcher Dr. Tom Brenna*

3

. . .

How Omega-3s Help Your Heart

During the Omega-3 Scientific Roundtable at our home, there was lively discussion about which organ of the body was most helped by the omega-3 effect. The heart won, with the brain a close second. A study by Harvard researchers, funded by the Centers for Disease Control and Prevention (CDC), estimates that eighty-four thousand deaths each year from heart disease could be prevented if people ate sufficient omega-3 EPA/DHA.[1] Remember my sticky stuff explanation of illness (page 5)? Cardiovascular disease is the result of plaque (sticky fats, sticky carbs, and other sticky biochemicals) that accumulates on the lining of the arteries. Omega-3s produce an anti-sticky-stuff effect within the blood vessels. Let's go into a typical blood vessel and see how this works.

HOW THE OMEGA-3 EFFECT CARES FOR YOUR HEART

Cardiovascular disease is the number one cause of death and disability in humans. Simply speaking, the cardiovascular system gets sick because two bad things happen:

• The blood vessel walls get stiff.
• The blood vessel lining—the endothelium—collects plaque and gets rough.

Stiff and sticky blood vessels (often from omega-3 insufficiency) lead to clots and high blood pressure. Soft and flexible blood vessels (omega-3 sufficiency) lead to normal blood flow and blood pressure.

Here are the six main things that can go wrong with your heart and how omega-3s can help make them right.

Heart Disease	The Omega-3 Heart Effect
• Your blood vessels get stiff, causing high blood pressure.	• Blood vessels are flexible, lowering high blood pressure.[2]
• The electrical system in your heart misfires. This is known as an arrhythmia.	• Heartbeat is steady and efficient. Lowers risk of sudden cardiac death.
• Blood vessels throughout your body, especially in your heart and brain, clog, resulting in coronary thrombosis or stroke.	• Blood consistency (clotting ability) is just right.
• The lining of your blood vessels, the endothelium, gets rough and worn, called inflammation.	• The lining of blood vessels is smooth. Less sticky stuff accumulates. Endothelial "pharmacy" dispenses natural internal "medicines."
• Fats stick to endothelium; plaque builds up, obstructing blood flow. This is called atherosclerosis.	• Plaque buildup is reduced. Existing plaques more stable; less likely to break off, causing stroke.
• Heart muscle weakens and fails, known as heart failure.	• Heart life is stronger, longer.

"You're only as healthy as your blood vessels" is one of the top medical truisms. That makes sense because the blood vessels supply every organ in the body. Let's go inside your arteries to see how omega-3s keep them wide open. I believe this is one of the biggest medical breakthroughs in the past decade.

MEET DR. NO

Did you know that your endothelium, the lining of your blood vessels, is the largest hormone-secreting organ in your body? I call it your personal pharmacy, where you make your own medicines. If you were to open up all your blood vessels and lay them out flat, they would occupy a surface larger than several tennis courts. The billions of cells that line your arteries don't just sit there; they do something. Inside your endothelial pharmacy are

• medicines that lower the "highs": high blood pressure and high cholesterol;
• medicines that raise the "lows": antidepressants;
• medicines that heal your hurts: anti-inflammatories.

The lining of your arteries contains metabolically active cells (like millions of microscopic medicine bottles) that help the arteries stay healthy, like a highway with a built-in maintenance system to keep the surface smooth. At present, twenty-three known biochemicals are secreted by the endothelium. For example, these cells secrete a built-in biochemical called nitric oxide (NO), which acts as a vasodilator to help the vascular highways (arteries) automatically widen during rush hour traffic (e.g., when your heart pumps harder during exercise) to let blood flow more smoothly. A friend of mine, Dr. Lou Ignarro, was corecipient of a Nobel Prize in 1998 for discovering the effects of NO. That's why I call him Dr. NO.

In the same way that feeding a maintenance crew better food would make them better able to care for the pavement surface of a highway, omega-3s boost endothelial nitric oxide and feed the endothelium to keep it smooth and help it operate efficiently. My simple explanation: omega-3s help keep sticky stuff off the lining of your blood vessels.

Endothelial dysfunction is the basis of most cardiovascular disease.[3] Consider omega-3 EPA/DHA your own live-in heart doctor, floating through your bloodstream, stopping to make a house call where needed. Omega-3s feed your endothelial pharmacy to keep it open 24/7.

KEEP YOUR PHARMACY OPEN

Keeping your pharmacy open is the key to heart health. Notice in the upper illustration at right how sufficient omega-3s keep the blood cells from sticking together so the blood can flow smoothly and how they keep plaque from collecting at the top of the medicine bottles so they can open. In the lower illustration, with omega-3 insufficiency, the blood cells clump, and the medicine bottles can't open because of the sticky stuff.

The reason heart doctors make such a big deal about keeping your arteries flexible is that the less stiff your arteries are, the longer your heart lasts. There's a new ultrasound noninvasive test that measures artery stiffness. It's called the systemic arterial compliance (SAC) test.

Remember, as vessels get stiff (high blood pressure), the heart has to work harder to force blood through stiffer arteries, and eventually the heart pump fails. In a fascinating study, heart researchers gave thirty-eight people with stiff arteries and high blood levels of sticky fats (called dyslipidemia) fish oil supplements for seven weeks: twelve got 3000 mg (3 grams) per day of EPA; twelve got 3000 mg per day of DHA; and fourteen got a placebo. Those in both groups taking fish oil supplements showed less arterial stiffness at the end of the seven-week period.

Endothelial Pharmacy OPEN

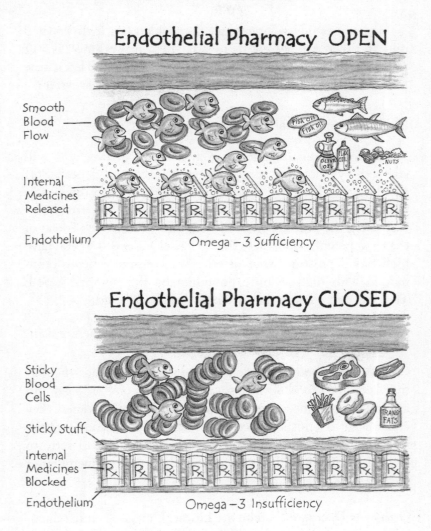

Smooth Blood Flow

Internal Medicines Released

Endothelium

Omega-3 Sufficiency

Endothelial Pharmacy CLOSED

Sticky Blood Cells

Sticky Stuff

Internal Medicines Blocked

Endothelium

Omega-3 Insufficiency

Systemic arterial compliance increased 36 percent in the EPA-treated group and 27 percent in the DHA-treated group, but there was no change in the placebo group.[4] Wow! Eat more fish oil, get less stiff. Arteries like that!

In another study, volunteers ate the stickiest fats, hydrogenated oils, and their arteries got more stiff.[5] Remember, illness is stiff tissues, wellness (the omega-3 effect) is soft tissues. This is true for all systems of the body, especially the cardiovascular system.

Omega-3s Help Lower High Blood Pressure

High blood pressure results from arteries' getting stiff and stressed. By helping to keep sticky stuff (excess fat deposits) off the lining of the blood vessels, omega-3s help keep the vessels more flexible.[6] Cardiologists believe omega-3s soften arteries by increasing the production of nitric oxide (NO), which is one of the most potent vasodilators (blood vessel wideners). If you have high blood pressure, your arteries are constantly being bombarded with high-pressure pounding by the pumped blood. They can't get the rest they need between heartbeats.

Omega-3s Keep Your Blood from Getting Too Thick

Omega-3s are known as membrane molecules. That's the way they keep the blood flowing smoothly. When omega-3s get into any cell membrane, especially the blood cell membranes, they create what scientists call cellular fluidity. This means that the more flexible or "fluid" the cell is, the better it is able to perform its healthy functions. In contrast, the stiffer the cell membranes are, the sicker the tissue.

Omega-3s Decrease Platelet Stickiness. Omega-3s attach themselves to other blood cells called platelets and make them behave the way they should. Platelets are millions of microscopic cells that clump together and clot when you get a cut. But sometimes platelets get their signals crossed and clot *inside* the vessel.[7]

There is a continuous clotting/anticlotting dance going on in the bloodstream. A chemical called thromboxane, produced by platelets in the blood, causes the platelets to clump together. To keep clots from forming where they shouldn't, for instance, in an artery in your brain or heart, the lining of your blood vessels produces a chemical called prostacyclin, which regulates blood clotting, balancing the clotting effects of the prostaglandins. After all, neither too easy clotting nor too easy bleeding is good for the body. Doctors sometimes prescribe a daily baby aspirin or a prescription anticoagulant to keep platelets from sticking together, although a diet high in omega-3s is a safer, more natural way to promote a healthy blood-clotting balance. Omega-3 EPA/DHA helps keep this balance.

Omega-3s Help Lower Lipids

To keep the omega-3 effect flowing, shall we say, let's return to protecting your endothelial pharmacy.

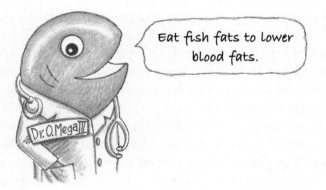

Cholesterol Confusion Clarified. The two normal fats in the blood are cholesterol and triglycerides, the ones your doctor measures when ordering a lipid panel. But oil (blood fats) and water don't mix. So, to make these fats soluble, blood proteins wrap snakelike around these fats, forming a blood-soluble compound called a lipoprotein. These LDL (low-density lipoprotein)

cholesterol compounds are like ferryboats transporting fats to receptors (docks) on tissues. (There are actually two lipoprotein ferryboats, one carrying cholesterol and the other triglycerides.) When the lipid-laden ferryboat arrives at the dock, such as the endothelium of the blood vessels, they deposit their tissue-building cargo, such as cholesterol passengers, onto the dock. Yet suppose the ferryboat is overloaded with excess sticky blood fats from that 16-ounce steak you scarfed down. The wobbly boat crashes into the dock (tissues) and dumps the excess sticky fats, which clump up on the dock as plaque.

Two healthful rescue efforts occur. Along comes a ferryboat with Captain HDL (high-density lipoprotein), who quickly mops up the mess and removes the excess cholesterol dumped on the docks before it has a chance to pile up and damage anything. The second helper is omega-3s, which make the docks stronger and the surface of the docks less sticky so that the excess cholesterol doesn't clump to form plaque.

Many consumers are confused about "good cholesterol" and "bad cholesterol." Here's more science made simple. Cholesterol is good; otherwise the body wouldn't naturally make it. It's one of the top fats for building brain tissue and making hormones. But when blood cholesterol levels get *too high* or the molecules get damaged (oxidized), some of the cholesterol molecules become too sticky, or "bad." The same is true for the other blood fat your doctor measures, triglycerides. These are normal, healthy fat molecules that act like ferryboats carrying fat nutrients to tissues. But if triglyceride levels get *too high,* they become sticky and their excess becomes "bad."

New insights suggest it's the number of small-particle cholesterol LDL complexes that are most damaging to the endothelial lining. Omega-3 supplements decrease the accumulation of sticky fats, triglycerides and small-particle LDL, that wriggle their way into arterial walls and make them stiff.[8]

LDL cholesterol, contrary to popular opinion, is not really a bad molecule, since without it your body, especially your brain, wouldn't work well. It's the excess of a particular heart-unhealthy type of LDL molecule called small-particle LDL that makes it behave badly. LDL cholesterol is considered a marker, meaning a risk factor. High LDL cholesterol is simply a red flag that alerts the doctor (and the patient) that you need extra help. It is not a life sentence that you're going to get heart disease, nor is a low or normal LDL a license to indulge, since half the people who have heart attacks have normal cholesterol.

The omega-3 effect on cholesterol is still being studied. Omega-3s may not lower cholesterol, but they do make cholesterol molecules behave so that they become less sticky and nourish the tissues instead of harming them.

In the United States we don't have a health care system; we have a disease care system. There is a paradigm shift among health care providers, meaning a change in thinking about disease. Many are moving beyond the cholesterol-centered view of cardiovascular disease to the inflammation-triggering cause. They are moving from the "low fat" viewpoint to the "right fat" viewpoint. That right fat is fish oil fat. This shift is also happening among health care consumers, who are asking, "Doctor, what can I *do*?" instead of "Doctor, what can I *take*?"

Omega-3s Help Stabilize Arterial Plaques

When plaque builds up on the walls of the arteries, it can do two deadly things:

- A piece of it can break off, travel downstream, and lodge in a small coronary artery or a vessel in the brain, causing a heart attack or stroke.
- It can stiffen the walls of arteries so much that they can't expand (hardening of the arteries). This raises blood pressure and lowers blood flow.

Omega-3s (EPA/DHA) stabilize plaques so they are less likely to loosen and break off.[9] These effects are why I like to call omega-3s artery conditioners.

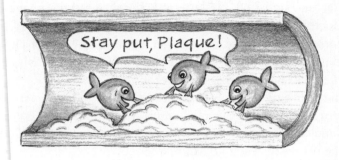

Omega-3s Lower Triglycerides. The Physicians' Health Study, a twenty-year study of twenty-two thousand male physicians, found that the heart attack rate rose proportional to a rising blood level of triglycerides.[10] The most relevant finding was that sudden death due to heart attack in these participants decreased proportionally with the increase in omega-3 EPA/DHA blood levels. When omega-3 levels in red blood cell membranes were measured, those with the highest levels had a 70 percent reduction in the rate of death from cardiac arrhythmias.

Researchers conclude that omega-3s exert a lipid-lowering effect by both decreasing the liver's production of triglycerides and increasing the body's ability to eliminate an excess of these sticky fats. More doctors are coming to believe that lowering high blood triglyceride levels and achieving a lower ratio of ARA (an omega-6 fat) to EPA may be as important as lowering high cholesterol.

There is another way omega-3s may help lessen the effect of high cholesterol on arterial health: by increasing the LDL particle size. It's the small particles of cholesterol that worm their way into the lining and walls of arteries, depositing cholesterol and making them sticky and stiff. Because the science on how omega-3s help regulate excess cholesterol is confusing and often conflicting, I asked the cardiovascular researcher Dr. William Harris to clarify it. His science-made-simple explanation: "Omega-3s help keep the endothelial lining smooth so excess cholesterol can't stick to it." This description validates my sticky stuff explanation of illness.

NEW RESEARCH: OMEGA-3S DECREASE STICKY STUFF IN BLOOD VESSELS

A 2011 analysis of studies involving seven hundred people showed that supplementation with omega-3s lowered the blood level of homocysteine, a by-product of protein metabolism.[11] By some biochemical quirk, high levels of homocysteine act like sticky stuff, which damages the lining of the blood vessels and increases the tendency of blood to clot too fast. Many cardiologists measure the blood level of homocysteine because a person's risk of heart disease goes up if their homocysteine level gets too high. High homocysteine levels may also increase the risk of cognitive decline and Alzheimer's disease, diseases of excess sticky stuff accumulation in the brain.

Omega-3s Help Heartbeats

People, especially athletes, who enjoy a slightly lower resting heart rate (50–60 beats per minute) tend to have healthier hearts. Research shows that people who eat more omega-3s tend to have lower resting heart rates.[12] Add to this the fact that dietary omega-3s can blunt the heart-rate-increasing effects of stress hormones. Imagine the longevity-enhancing effects of a lower number of beats per minute. This translates into millions of heartbeats saved, less wear and tear on the heart, and perhaps a longer life.

The heart is a strong muscle with electrical currents going through it, and it has a built-in pulse generator called a pacemaker. That pacemaker automatically fires around 60–90 times per minute. It fires faster when you need it to work harder; for example, when you run. But sometimes the pacemaker misfires. This is called an arrhythmia. If it stops firing or fires wildly, the heart can stop pumping and cause sudden cardiac death. Research shows that omega-3s help regulate the pacemaker, keeping it from misfiring.[13] In the famous GISSI study of eleven thousand patients, Italian scientists gave omega-3 EPA/DHA fish oil (850 mg per day in an EPA to DHA ratio of 1.2:1) to one group of heart attack patients but not to another, and then followed these patients for over three years. The omega-3 EPA/DHA group had a 45 percent lower rate of sudden death from heart stoppage, and a 10 percent lower rate of death from all other causes, compared to the other group.[14] Wow! Pass the fish oil, please. This study, published in the prestigious medical journal *The Lancet*, made omega-3s famous.

Young Hearts Love Omega-3s

Cardiovascular disease, especially high blood pressure, can begin in childhood, decades before any symptoms of heart problems are likely to appear. A study of more than three thousand young Americans (15–34 years of age) who died of other causes between 1987 and 1994 revealed that young children on unhealthy diets can have early signs of cardiovascular disease.[15] About 20 percent of the 15–19-year-old adolescents already showed fatty streaks in their abdominal aortas. About 40 percent of the 30–34-year-olds also showed these fatty streaks. Researchers recommended that cardiovascular disease prevention begin in childhood or at least by early adolescence.

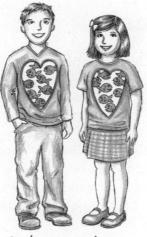

Help young hearts
grow healthier

Omega-3s can lower high blood pressure in overweight teens. Teens given 1500 mg (1.5 grams) of EPA/DHA had lower systolic blood pressure by an average of 3.8 and diastolic 2.6.[16] Even slight decreases in blood pressure over a long period of time can lessen the load on the heart. You can help young hearts grow healthier by feeding your children more omega-3 EPA/DHA.

EAT MORE FISH, ENJOY MORE HEART HEALTH

For a healthier heart, go fish! In a famous study called the Nurses' Health Study, Harvard researchers studied five thousand female nurses who had diabetes. There was a striking correlation: the more fish they ate, the lower their risk of developing heart disease. The nurses who consumed fish once a week had a 40 percent lower risk; those eating fish five times a week had a 64 percent lower risk.[17]

THE TALE OF TWO FATS

Remember my explanation of cardiovascular disease: you put sticky fats in your mouth, you get sticky stuff in your heart. I began to advise my patients to eat more omega-3s after a close friend of mine suffered a massive heart attack and almost died after gorging at a steakhouse. That near-tragedy prompted me to study how differently the fats from fish and the fats from steak behave in the bloodstream. Let's follow a typical supermarket steak and a wild salmon fillet and see how one can make you sick and fat, and the other can help you be well and lean.

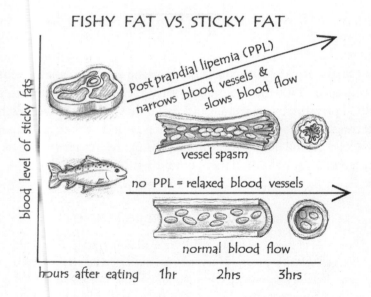

FISHY FAT VS. STICKY FAT

blood level of sticky fats

Post prandial lipemia (PPL) narrows blood vessels & slows blood flow

vessel spasm

no PPL = relaxed blood vessels

normal blood flow

hours after eating   1hr   2hrs   3hrs

Sticky Steak. You begin to scarf down a steak, prized for its marbling. (It's noteworthy that during autopsies pathologists label marbling in muscle as "pathologic infiltration of fat.") A few hours after this high-fat meal, triglyceride levels go up along with another sticky substance called fibrinogen, which is like a fishnet of chemicals that help your blood clot. This is called postprandial lipemia (PPL), the medical term for a high level of sticky fats after a meal that float through your bloodstream, gradually clumping together and forming blood clots. PPL can decrease endothelial function. The endothelium of your blood vessels reacts to this sticky stuff by going into spasm, or vasoconstriction, in which blood vessels get narrower and blood slows to a sludgelike flow. A traffic jam occurs inside your vessels. Not only do the cars (red blood cells) clump together but the vessel highway gets narrower. This can lead to a heart attack or stroke. Cardiologists call this the steakhouse syndrome.

Smooth Seafood. Unlike those sticky fats in steak that narrow blood vessels and slow blood flow, fishy fats relax blood vessels and speed blood flow, like a highway widening during rush hour and traffic flowing more smoothly. After a person eats heart-healthy

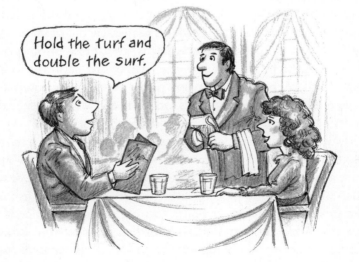

omega-3 EPA/DHA foods, PPL doesn't occur. Because these sea-foods have soft and flexible fats, blood vessels don't go into spasm. The effect of dietary fats on vascular reactivity is becoming a topic of interest for cardiovascular health.[18]

People who take fish oil supplements experience PPL less often after they eat a high-fat meal. So having a continuous high level of omega-3s may blunt the sticky stuff effect of an occasional indulgence in steak.[19] (See more about PPL, page 127.)

HEART HEALTH QUESTIONS YOU MAY HAVE

Omega-3s Plus Prescription Anticoagulants

What if my doctor prescribes blood thinners such as aspirin, Plavix, or warfarin (e.g., Coumadin)? Can I still take omega-3 EPA/DHA supplements?

Yes, you can, and you should. The medical practice of blood thinning, substantiated by science, maintains that if you slightly decrease the tendency of your blood to clot, you'll suffer fewer heart attacks and strokes. These drugs lessen the tendency for blood to clot by different mechanisms from those of omega-3s. Omega-3 EPA/DHA regulates the level of the natural proclotting chemical thromboxane (see pages 46–47). And omega-3s make red blood cell membranes more flexible, which lessens the tendency of blood cells to clump and clot too fast.

If you need anticoagulant therapy, the dilemma for your doctor is to thin your blood just enough to reduce your risk of having a brain artery stroke or a clot in your coronary arteries but not too much to cause you to bleed excessively. Do you eat extra fish oil, take prescription drugs, or both? Current medical practice is to prescribe a blood-thinning drug and then measure your blood-clotting tendency by a blood test called INR (International Normalized Ratio). This test is most accurate when taken while you eat your usual diet. If you eat seafood and/or take fish oil supplements as part of your usual diet, the INR will reflect this dietary practice, and your doctor can adjust your dosage accordingly. When you are taking prescription blood thinners, you must be *consistent* in your dietary omega-3 intake and always inform your doctor if you make drastic changes in how much daily omega-3 you eat.

The dose of omega-3s recommended for most people, 500–1000 mg per day, shouldn't increase risk of bleeding. Properly monitored, even eating 6 ounces of oily fish as often as four times a week (about 1000 mg omega-3 EPA/DHA per day) does not cause abnormal bleeding.

I thoroughly reviewed the medical literature on this concern. Studies showed that a moderate consumption (2000–5000 mg per day) of omega-3s did not appear to increase the risk of bleeding, even if taken with aspirin or warfarin.

General expert conclusions point to no scientific evidence that therapeutic doses of omega-3s significantly increase bleeding, and the medical benefits of omega-3s more than outweigh the theoretical risks of increased bleeding. The bottom line is to follow the American Heart Association guideline that because of concerns about excessive anticoagulant effect, people taking more than 3000 mg (3 grams) of omega-3 EPA/DHA per day should do so only under a physician's supervision. See related information on bleeding concerns in the section Omega-3s: Nutritional Armor for the Military, page 145, and what scientists say about omega-3s and bleeding.[20]

Perhaps science will soon confirm what some omega-3 researchers suspect: fish oil is a safer anticoagulant than prescription medications. The February 2012 issue of the *Harvard Health Letter* reported research revealing that prescription anticoagulants, especially Coumadin, accounted for nearly 50 percent of emergency hospitalizations for drug side effects. Most of these hospitalizations were from excessive bleeding.

Fish Oil Plus Cholesterol-Lowering Medications

*My doctor prescribed a statin medicine to lower
my high cholesterol. Should I also be taking fish oil?*
Some people have quirks in cholesterol metabolism, causing
their liver to make too much of this sticky stuff. So they have to
take cholesterol-lowering medications called statins. Here's where
omega-3 EPA science shines. The 2007 JELIS (Japan EPA Lipid
Intervention Study) research reported in the British medical journal *The Lancet* found that omega-3 EPA helps statin drugs work
better. In this study people who took EPA in addition to statins
had 20 percent fewer major heart problems than those who took
statins alone.[21] Many doctors now prescribe fish oil supplements
when they prescribe cholesterol-lowering statin drugs.

The JELIS found that EPA supplementation reduced heart
attacks, improved angina, and reduced deaths due to heart
attacks. This large-scale clinical trial involved 4,900 doctors and
18,645 patients with hypercholesterolemia and a mean age of 61
years, randomly selected to receive either 1800 mg EPA plus statins,
statins only, or a placebo. The group that received EPA plus statins
experienced 20 percent fewer heart attacks compared with those
who received statins alone. The conclusion of the study: statins
may increase the blood levels of proinflammatory ARA, but the
anti-inflammatory effects of EPA balance these. Based on this
science, many cardiologists prescribe high doses of omega-3s
before, or at least in addition to, statin therapy.

One of the largest studies on the use of omega-3s to lower the
mortality rate from cardiovascular disease (CVD), the GISSI
study (see page 52), showed that omega-3 fish oil supplements
lowered the risk of death from CVD, but cholesterol-lowering
statins did not.[22] Whether or not statin medications lower the
mortality rate from CVD is currently a subject of debate among
cardiologists and awaits more study.

Heart-Healthy Kids

How can I explain the eat-more-omega-3s concept to my kids?

Try this: Omega-3s help the blood flow smoothly like kids on a slippery waterslide. They wriggle their way into the lining of the blood vessels to keep them smooth and soft. Unlike those sticky fats that stick together in your bloodstream and pile up on the

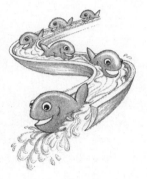

walls of the vessels like a waterslide without water, omega-3s keep things smooth. Because they are a "smoothie" fat instead of a sticky fat, your body likes them.

Heart Unhealthy Husband

Dr. Bill, I love my husband, but I'm frustrated. He just won't take care of his heart. His family tree is littered with early deaths from heart disease. He already has high blood pressure. He hates fish and thinks fish oil is flaky. How can I help him?

Readers, my answer may surprise you: The best way to a man's heart is through his penis. Even though I am stretching the science a bit, it usually takes such shock statements to get men to make healthy changes.

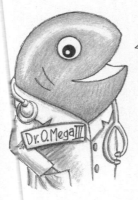

Men, did you know that the better you take care of your heart, the better your erections will be? In fact, many men visit the doctor because they've experienced erectile dysfunction (ED), and the doctor discovers underlying cardiovascular disease, such as high blood pressure or a weak heart. The reason that penis problems are often the first clue to heart disease is that the health of both these organs depends on the health of their blood vessels.

When you eat too much of the wrong fats and not enough of the fats that keep your blood flowing more smoothly, you put yourself at risk for endothelial dysfunction (ED). Because getting and maintaining a healthy erection depends on your blood vessels' being smooth and wide open, the ED of the heart can lead to the other ED.

So, guys, the safest medicine for your penis is the same as the safest one for your heart: the omega-3 oils found in seafood and fish oil supplements.

Feeling Fine

Doctor, I feel fine. Why should I take fish oil supplements?

Here's a shocking statistic: 50 percent of sudden cardiac deaths occur in people who "feel fine" and have no prior history of heart disease.

In fact, the 90 percent reduction in the rate of sudden cardiac death in people who took adequate omega-3s is one of the highlights of cardiovascular research. Omega-3s are not only one of the top therapeutic nutrients but also, in my opinion and that of many other doctors, the number one nutraceutical in preventive medicine.[23]

WHAT'S IN YOUR ARTERIES ?

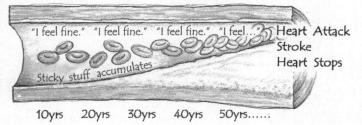

Eating sufficient omega-3s may have these heart-healthy effects:
• Reduced risk of heart attacks
• Better blood pressure
• Lower incidence of angina
• Stabilized vessel plaque
• Less risk of sudden cardiac death

For optimal omega-3 effect on cardiovascular health:
• Eat at least 12 ounces of oily seafood per week, and/or take at least 1000 mg of omega-3 EPA/ DHA fish oil supplements daily.
• Eat more seafood, less meat.
• Give yourself an oil change: eat more omega-3 oils.

4

. . .

How Omega-3s Build Smarter
Brains and Better Moods

Besides being heart-healthy, omega-3s help build brighter brains. The brain needs omega-3s as much as the heart does, perhaps even more so. After all, the brain is one of the most vascular organs in the body. Which organ requires the most flexible, fluid multitasking and the fastest response? The brain. Which fat has these same qualities? Omega-3 EPA/DHA. That's why omega-3s and brain function are perfect partners in health.

Omega-3s help improve the Ds:

- Mood disorders: OCD (obsessive-compulsive disorder), BPD (bipolar disorder), and other Ds like depression
- Dementia, Alzheimer's disease
- Childhood Ds: ADHD/ADD

OMEGA-3S ARE SMART FATS

Your brain is 60 percent fat, so if somebody calls you a fathead, take it as a compliment. It's interesting that perhaps our most important organ also has the largest proportion of fat. While many different

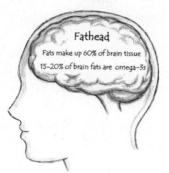

Fathead
Fats make up 60% of brain tissue
15–20% of brain fats are omega-3s

fats make up the brain, omega-3 DHA alone makes up 15–20 per-cent of the brain's fat. Many fad diets want us to eat less of this prime structural component of the brain.

The three hardest-working tissues in the body, the brain/retina, the testes, and the heart, are highest in omega-3 content. The human brain is the top performer, using 20 percent of the total food energy consumed (chimps use only 13 percent), even though its weight is only 1–2 percent of total body weight.

Research shows that people with the highest blood levels of omega-3 DHA display the best brain performance. The higher the omega-3 blood levels (DHA), the higher the brain test scores. Analysis of the brains of people with various nerve diseases, such as multiple sclerosis and macular degeneration, found that they had plenty of omega-6s but low levels of omega-3s in their brain tissue.

At least once a day I remind my patients: right-fat instead of low-fat diets are best for the body and brain. This sounds like, shall we say, a no-brainer. Since omega-3 DHA is one of the top fats in the brain, you need to eat more omega-3s. This chapter explains how these omegas work to help you think better and feel happier.

When addressing military brass on why omega-3s could help combat troops make quick decisions and moves, Captain Joseph Hibbeln, MD, summed up, "When you change your fats, you change your brain."

There are three important brain structures:

- The brain cell (called a neuron), especially the membrane
- The nerve extending from the neuron, called an axon
- The connections at the end of the neuron, called synapses

Omega-3s make each of these three components healthier so that your thoughts can fire faster.

OMEGAS BUILD BETTER BRAIN CELLS

Remember, omega-3s strengthen cell membranes and make them function better. "You're only as healthy as your cell membranes" goes double for brain cell membranes, which work harder than most other cells of the body. Just as a processor powers a computer, omegas act as the "Intel Inside" in the biochemical programming of the brain. Omegas provide nutrients needed for brain growth, brain tissue maintenance and repair, and brain food for all that nerve traffic that is working 24/7. Science agrees: Experimental animals and humans whose diets were deficient in omega-3 fats or who had low omega-3 blood levels were found to have smaller brains than com-

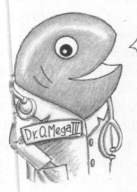

I help brain cells make the right connections.

parison groups. Omega-3s nourish the brain. Here's how the neurology researcher Dr. Tom Brenna explained the omega-3 effect to me: "Nerve traffic is like a wave in the sea traveling down the nerve cell membrane. Omega-3s act like tiny fish using their fins to assist the waves of nerve energy to travel faster."[1]

OMEGA-3S ARE MEMBRANE MOLECULES

The two top omega-3s, EPA and DHA, help build the structural components of the cell membranes, and like the processor inside a computer, they help the biochemical machinery of the cell membranes work better. EPA and DHA are the brain brothers: DHA helps the structure and EPA helps the functioning of brain tissue. Omega-3s are appropriately called cell conditioners. In the same way as hair conditioner makes your hair soft and flexible, omega-3 EPA/DHA makes the cell membranes more flexible.

OMEGA-3S MAKE MYELIN WORK BETTER

The long fibers (axons) extending from a brain cell—like tentacles from an octopus—are coated with a fatty sheath called myelin (white matter), which acts like insulation on electrical wires and makes the electrical messages in the brain travel faster (myelination). Myelin is 70–80 percent fat, made mostly of the stiff saturated fats and cholesterol (perfectly suited to these particular tissues). Just as frayed insulation on electrical wires slows electrical impulses, damaged myelin causes thoughts to be fuzzy, forgetful, and slower, and makes muscle movements uncoordinated. For example, multiple sclerosis is a debilitating disease in which the myelin insulation on the nerve fibers becomes frayed. Studies have shown that blood levels of omega-3s were low in patients with multiple sclerosis, and that omega-3 supplementation can be effective in battling the disease.[2] The psychiatrist Dr. George Bartzokis describes myelin as "insulation on steroids" because it increases both the speed of transmission and the bandwidth.[3]

Which nerve cell would you like?

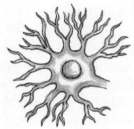 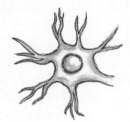

| Omega-3 sufficiency | Omega-3 insufficiency |
| (more connections) | (fewer connections) |

Myelination increases the speed and the amount of information that can travel across nerve fibers at one time. In Internet terminology, we would call this "expanding the bandwidth." We think faster, innovate, multitask, and retain knowledge mainly because of myelin. In effect, myelin upgrades the nerve circuits to process information more efficiently. In fact, an increasingly popular explanation of neurological and even psychiatric disorders is thought to be dysfunction in myelination.

How Omegas Make Myelin. The healthier your myelin, the better your brain behaves and performs. My quest to discover the omega-3 effect on myelin prompted me to consult Dr. Bartzokis, a professor of psychiatry at UCLA and one of the world's top myelin researchers. Here's what I learned.[4] Hovering around the nerve cell tissues (gray matter) are millions of myelin-making cells called oligodendrocytes. (You made more myelin by just pronouncing their name!) Let's call them O-cells for short. These spiderlike cells spin a web of myelin around the nerve, like bubble-wrapping a precious glass. The more wrapping, the more protection. When myelin wears out—gets frayed—these O-cells click into the repair-and-protect mode, and these cells secrete more myelin. Those tiny myelin-making O-cells are what make human brains smarter. We make much more myelin than, say, a chimpanzee does. In fact, Dr. Bartzokis describes humans as "myelin beings."

One day I was playing catch with my eighteen-month-old grandson, Landon. He seemed to have a talent for throwing a ball accurately. "Aha, future major league pitcher," I thought, as I clicked into my myelin-making mode. I realized that the more we played catch, the more he threw the ball, the more his O-cells cranked out myelin. That's part of why practice makes perfect. I imagined that every time he threw the ball, he was wrapping more and more of his nerves in myelin. Playing catch, going fishing, and making myelin could be this little kid's pathway to becoming a star pitcher.

Remember, omegas feed O-cells. So each time you savor your salmon or take a fish oil supplement, imagine you're making more myelin. O-cells are the active kids of the brain cells. O-cells produce three times their weight in myelin each day. During myelin-making the O-cells use more than twice the energy of other brain cells, and their use of nutrients to synthesize brain fats is six times as high. This high metabolic rate makes these myelin-producing cells more susceptible to oxidation. The anti-oxidant or anti-inflammatory effect of omega-3s on the O-cells prevents the oxidation of myelin. In simple language, high metabolic stress could make a metabolic mess of the myelin-making cells and lead to frayed insulation (damaged myelin). Omega-3s protect nerve tissue by producing biochemicals appropriately called neuroprotectins. A way to remember how omega-3s protect brain cells from oxidation: one O (omega-3s) protects another O (the O-cells) against oxidation.

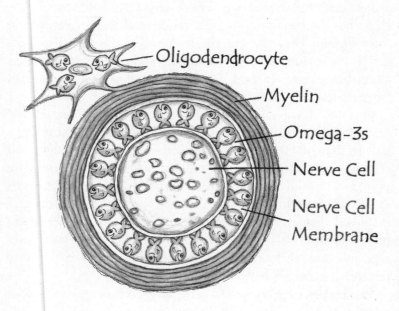

Oligodendrocyte
Myelin
Omega-3s
Nerve Cell
Nerve Cell Membrane

Structurally, myelin is a mixed blessing. On the one hand, its high percentage of fat makes it more receptive to nutritional and perhaps pharmaceutical interventions. On the other hand, fat tissue is more vulnerable to toxins, disease, disintegration, and nutritional deficiencies. Research shows that an omega-3 deficiency can lead to damaged myelin, which can be reversed in people who take omega-3 supplements.[5] Since myelin is the neurological weak link, it makes sense to eat more omega-3s to make and repair myelin. Myelin production seems to peak around age 45 and may decline thereafter unless we nourish and protect it.

The Hummingbird Story. An important omega-3 effect that my expert consultants pointed out was that tissues that work the hardest, such as the brain and eyes, have the highest concentration of omega-3s. In fact, some of the hardest working tissues in nature, the pectoral muscles of the hummingbird (which are half the weight of the bird) have extraordinarily high levels of omega-3s (more than 20 percent), as high as the percentage in the human eye.[6] One reason is that the flexibility of those "tall guy" omega-3s supports the rapid flexing of those energetic muscles. Omega-3s are potent antioxidants that protect these hardworking tissues.

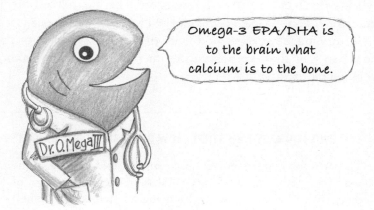

OMEGA-3S FEED BRAIN MESSENGERS

Omega-3 EPA/DHA acts like the brain's communication director. The junction or gap between two nerve cells (neurons) trying to communicate with each other is called a synapse, from the Greek "to bind together." The neurons have some of the highest concentration of DHA of any tissue of the body. Here's how neurons communicate with one another. A neuron releases neurotransmitters, biochemical messengers that carry information like high-speed ferryboats from one neuron across the synapse to another neuron. On the receiver neuron's cell membranes are microscopic receptor sites into which the neurotransmitters must fit. Think of the receptor sites as custom-made docks that fit the arriving neurotransmitter ferryboats. Omega-3s feed these ferryboats, or brain messengers, enabling them to travel faster and more efficiently; these malleable molecules work their way into the receptor sites and tweak them so that they can more effectively receive the messages.

If you don't eat enough omega-3s, three things can happen: the neurotransmitter ferryboats don't travel fast enough; the ferryboats don't fit into their respective docks; or the cell membranes can become loaded and clogged with the wrong fats (such as factory-made hydrogenated fats), distorting the shape of the docks so that the ferryboats won't fit into them, thus making docking more difficult.

AN EVOLUTIONARY FISH STORY: HOW OUR BRAINS GOT BIGGER

The neurology researcher Dr. Tom Brenna told me one of the most compelling fish stories validating the importance of omega-3s as the smart fat. Anthropologists increasingly believe omega-3s may be the biochemical basis for why human brains got bigger and humans got smarter. According to Professor Michael Crawford, director of the Institute of Brain Chemistry and Human Nutrition in London, after the migration of early humans from central to coastal areas and adaptation of their diet from plant food to seafood, the human brain tripled in weight from 1 to 3 pounds.[7] Dr. Crawford makes another point about the omega-3 effect: the brains of sea animals are proportionally much larger (weight of brain/weight of body) than the brains of land animals. Perhaps this would be a good fish story to tell schoolchildren to get them to eat more seafood.

OMEGA-3S IMPROVE VISION: SEAFOOD IS SEE FOOD

What's good for the brain is good for the eyes. Your ability to read this page is helped by the high concentration of DHA in your eyes. The back part of your eyes—the projection screen called the retina and macula, on which your lenses focus light— is simply an extension of your brain. So if omega-3 EPA/DHA is good for the brain, it would be good for the eyes, too. The usual illnesses of the aging eye, such as cataracts, age-related macular degeneration (ARMD), and glaucoma, could be caused by inflammation and an omega-3 deficiency. The retina has the highest tissue oxidation capacity (wear and tear) of any tissue in the body. Besides omega-3 oils, seafood contains other potent antioxidants, such as selenium and astaxanthin. So focus on go fish!

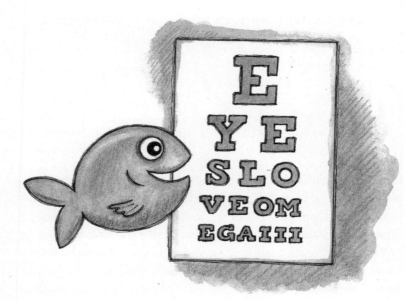

Because it's part of the brain, the retina of the eye has one of the highest concentrations of DHA in the body. The omega-3 smart fats feed the hyperactive cells of the retina, so named because these photoreceptor cells are so high functioning that they wear out quickly and need to be replaced almost daily by new cells. Tissues that have high metabolic energy are prone to oxidation (wear and tear). These cells are examples of what I call high-need cells, those that require a constant source of omega-3s to survive and thrive.

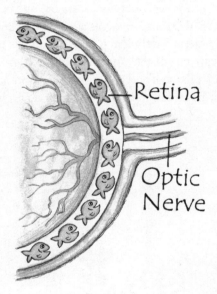

Omega-3s Help Keep Eyes Younger. Research reveals that people who take DHA in fish oil in combination with the antioxidant lutein have increased pigment density throughout the retina.[8] *Pigment density* is the term eye doctors use for the concentration of protective nutrients, mainly carotenoids, in the cells of the retina. These nutrients have powerful antioxidant properties, helping to mellow the wear and tear of sunlight photons striking sensitive retinal tissue. Macular pigments decline with age, eventually leading to ARMD, the leading cause of blindness in seniors. Again, science validates common sense. Retinal tissue is primarily fat (DHA) and blood vessels. As in other tissues, the protective omega effect is probably due both to its tissue-building properties and its antioxidant effects on retinal tissue.

SCIENCE SAYS: OMEGA-3 DHA IS EYE FOOD

Here's what research says about omega-3s for your vision:

- When doctors fed omega-3 DHA to premature babies, they developed better vision.
- Children whose mothers ate oily fish during pregnancy had better visual depth perception at age 3.5 years.[9]
- The higher the omega-3 DHA levels in mother's milk, the higher the visual acuity in her breast-fed infant.
- Infants fed formula supplemented with omega-3s showed improved visual function. The beneficial effect of omega-3s on visual development was most pronounced in preterm infants.
- Omega-3s have been found to help dry eyes, presumably by decreasing inflammation in the lacrimal glands and increasing the "oiliness" of tears.[10]
- Seniors who take fish oil have a lower incidence of age-related macular degeneration.[11]

OMEGA-3S ARE MOOD MELLOWERS

Smart patients and doctors are searching for healthier alternatives to prescription psychiatric drugs, especially in light of recent scientific exposés revealing that except for severe psychiatric illnesses, these risky medications may be no more effective than a placebo (sugar pill), and in many patients they can do more harm than good. Omega-3s to the rescue!

A depressing statistic that made headlines in the October 20, 2011, issue of USA Today: 12 percent of teens and 25 percent of adult women take prescription antidepressants. About 23 million U.S. adults suffer from mood disorders, or what I call the Ds: depression, obsessive-compulsive disorder (OCD), bipolar disorder (BPD), and so on. One reason I began prescribing omega-3 EPA/DHA in my medical practice is that it follows my general formula of practicing medicine: prescribe medicine based upon good sense and good science. Since mood disorders seem to be the result of misfiring or miswiring of neurotransmitters in the mood centers of the brain, and omega-3 EPA/DHA is the main structural and functional molecule of nerve firing and wiring, it seems logical that making sure the brain gets enough of these "happy molecules" should be a priority. Scientists agree.[12]

A meta-analysis of studies showed clear benefits of omega-3s for depression and bipolar disorder, leading the American Psychiatric Association to recommend a dosage greater than 1000 mg per day of EPA/DHA as an add-on for general treatment of mood disorders and possibly in addition to appropriate psychotropic drugs. Experts assembled by the Committee on Research on Psychiatric Treatments of the American Psychiatric Association reviewed the current research and concluded that omega-3 EPA/DHA showed significant benefits in the treatment of bipolar and major depression.[13] They also suggested that omega-3s may provide additional health benefits because of the prevalence of obesity and metabolic side effects of some psychotropic medications.

Psychiatric medicine teaches that depression is due in part to a biochemical imbalance, presumably of neurotransmitters like serotonin. While this neurotransmitter imbalance hypothesis remains unproven, preliminary studies suggest an omega-3 deficiency may be one of the biochemical imbalances in people with depression. Imbalances of omega-3s have been found in the red blood cell membranes of some depressed persons. This finding reinforces the reigning hypothesis that the basic defect in brain biochemistry of mood disorders is inflammation. Since omega-3s are powerful anti-inflammatories, that would explain how omega-3s affect depression by a different mechanism than do prescription antidepressants.

Omega-3s are called mood mellowers because they provide the food for hormones like serotonin and dopamine, which I like to call the "happy hormones" because they are associated with joy and calmness. A study of the brains of experimental animals that were given omega-3 supplements showed an increase in the number of dopamine receptors on their brain cells.

When you have an omega-3 deficiency, you get flaky skin — and a flaky brain.

—Joseph Hibbeln, MD

Omega-3s Protect the Brain. Omega-3s are neuroprotective against depression and other mood disorders. PET scans, radiology images that show brain activity, reveal that severely depressed patients suffer from shrinkage of the hippocampus, the area of the brain that controls memory and learning. Omega-3s from fish oil may benefit brain cell growth in this region. In contrast, diets low in omega-3s seem to destroy the brain's connective feelers, the synapses and dendrites, in the hippocampus. A 2011 study revealed that omega-3-deficient experimental animals suffer a reduced function of nerve cell receptors that facilitate healthy moods.[14]

EAT MORE OMEGA-3S, HANDLE STRESS BETTER

Perhaps the saying "worried sick" has a biological basis. High levels of stress hormones, or high cortisol levels, are another cause of brain shrinkage. Brain cells are overstimulated and literally wear out. This condition, called glucocorticoid neurotoxicity, can result in a variety of mood disorders. One of the neuroprotective functions of omega-3s is to protect the connections between brain cells from attack by high levels of stress hormones.

I agree with the opinion of Dr. Bill Lands on how seafood lessens the effects of stress: "The sea may give us food that lessens our overreactions to the stresses in our lives on land."[15]

Those researchers who have earned D degrees like MDs and PhDs really like omega-3s for helping their patients with illness Ds get better. Neurologists believe omega-3s fight depression by altering the brain's neurotransmitters, increasing serotonin receptors, and boosting dopamine levels in the "happy centers" of the brain, the frontal lobes. Mood disorders are thought to be a chemical imbalance of serotonin, dopamine, and other neurotransmitters, such as norepinephrine. Researchers generally agree that the role of EPA in alleviating mood disorders is primarily improving blood flow to the brain and decreasing inflammation of brain tissue.

The healthy fats found in oily seafood and fish oil supplements are becoming one of the most researched medicines for depression. Omega-3s help lower the highs (manic states) and raise the lows (depression). These "merry omegas" also help put a bit of a brain brake on people with impulsive and aggressive tendencies. (See section on military stress, page 145.)

Could Omega-3s Be Lifesaving? In 2009 I was a guest on a fishing expedition in Alaska. One of the other guests was the French physician and omega-3 researcher Dr. Thierry Lerond. I went fishing for some French connections between omega-3s and mental health. Dr. Lerond showed me the results of his study, which revealed that French soldiers who took omega-3 supplements were less likely to suffer psychiatric illnesses. When we met again, in September 2011, he shared with me that he had been invited to a NATO Operations Medical Conference to present his research to officers of the U.S. military.

The September 20, 2011, issue of *USA Today* showed the front-page headline, "Army Looking at How Fish Oil Might Reduce Suicides," referring to a study conducted by the noted omega-3 researcher Dr. Joseph Hibbeln of the National Institutes of Health and his colleagues that compared groups of eight hundred service members and found that those with the lowest levels of omega-3s were 62 percent more likely to commit suicide.[16]

BEHAVIORAL BRAIN CLAIMS

The results of what science says about omega-3s for psychiatric illnesses are often difficult to interpret because so many other therapies are going on simultaneously and patient reporting is highly subjective. So we're often left with what common sense says: Eat smarter fats, enjoy a better-behaved brain.

AN UPSET IMMUNE SYSTEM MAY CAUSE AN UPSET MIND

If you ask a psychiatrist what causes mood disorders, you're likely to get the explanation, "It's a chemical imbalance in the brain." An exciting new field called PNI, psychoneuroimmunology (how your brain and immune system connect), reveals that one of the root causes of these chemical imbalances is excessive inflammation in the body.[17] It follows that mood disorders are part of the epidemic in the spectrum of inflammatory disorders. Since omega-3s are potent anti-inflammatories, this new research helps explain why people who eat more seafood or take fish oil supplements enjoy happier moods.

A clue to the relation between omega-3s and the anti-inflammatory effect came from the discovery that depressed people tend to have higher levels of proinflammatory biochemicals called cytokines. The pieces of the depression puzzle started to fit together. Validating the omega-3 deficiency–inflammation–depression connection was another discovery: people with low blood levels of omega-3s also tend to have high levels of proinflammatory cytokines, and vice versa.

These findings go along with the discovery that both depressed people and those with chronic inflammatory diseases tend to have an omega-3 deficiency. Researchers discovered that an omega-6/omega-3 imbalance (excess omega-6s and insufficient omega-3s) leads to an exaggerated production of cytokines in response to stress. Eating more omega-3 EPA/DHA seems to modulate this inflammatory overreaction. Whether an omega-3 insufficiency is one of the causes of inflammatory imbalance and consequent mood disorders or just correlated with them remains to be proven.

OMEGAS IN MEDICAL SCHOOL

Medical students who had a higher blood level of omega imbalance (high omega-6/omega-3 ratio) showed higher inflammatory markers of stress during exams.

A 2011 study at Ohio State University College of Medicine showed that medical students who took omega-3 supplements suffered less anxiety and inflammation.[18]

OMEGA-3S HELP PREVENT ALZHEIMER'S DISEASE

In March 2011 I was playing golf with Dr. Vince Fortanasce, professor of neurology at the University of Southern California

School of Medicine and author of *The Anti-Alzheimer's Prescription*. Since this was a bad day for my golf score, I seized the opportunity to learn the latest scoop on Alzheimer's disease.

Dr. Fortanasce opened with, "Despite what you may read, there are currently no drugs that treat Alzheimer's once it occurs." I responded, "But, Vince, I know one of the most promising 'drugs' that may prevent or delay the onset of Alzheimer's, and perhaps even slow the progression a bit. Even though the science is not yet conclusive, and even a bit controversial, there is some promising research."

The science on omega-3 EPA/DHA as a brain function preserver is promising but not yet conclusive. Three of four clinical trials showed a small but significant benefit from omega-3s in people who were either at early stages of Alzheimer's disease or had a genetic risk factor for early-onset Alzheimer's.[19] It has been discovered that many Alzheimer's patients can't make enough DHA from the omega-3 found in plant foods, such as ALA. This seems to be due to a liver defect that prevents them from converting ALA to DHA. When researchers at the University of California, Irvine, examined liver tissue from patients with Alzheimer's disease, they found a genetic defect that diminishes the liver's ability to convert ALA to DHA. Also, brain tissue samples from patients with Alzheimer's showed low levels of DHA. Several studies, but not all, showed that a higher intake of fish, and therefore of EPA and DHA, reduces the risk of dementia.

The Zutphen Elderly Study, published in 2007, showed that people eating an average of 400 mg per day of omega-3 EPA/DHA from fish showed a much slower cognitive decline than people who did not eat enough omega-3s.[20]

Many neurological disorders, such as Parkinson's disease and Alzheimer's disease, are now put in the category of inflammatory disorders. The clue to this was research showing that the risk of autism, ADHD, Alzheimer's, and Parkinson's goes up as the level of omega-3s goes down. More and more top brain scientists are coming to the conclusion that Alzheimer's disease, like so many of the other Ds, is at least partly caused by inflammation. That's why I lump it with other -itis illnesses and call it cognitivitis. Continuous inflammation in the brain causes accumulation of sticky stuff called amyloid deposits, which are deposited into the tissue. These then stimulate the immune system, which misinterprets this tissue as "foreign" and attacks it. Since omega-3s are potent anti-inflammatories, it makes sense to eat them to protect brain tissue from excessive wear and tear and to potentially help in repair.

NEUROLOGICAL QUESTIONS YOU MAY HAVE

Fish Oil Plus Prescription Drugs

So many of my friends are taking antidepressants. Would seafood and fish oil take the place of these prescription psychiatric drugs?

One of the leading theories of the root cause of many of the brain Ds, like depression and OCD, is that the keys (e.g., serotonin) don't fit the locks (receptors), or there are not enough keys to fill the locks. Theoretically, selective serotonin reuptake inhibitors (SSRIs), the most frequently prescribed class of mood-altering drugs, do increase the number of keys to fill the locks. Brain researchers believe that omega-3 EPA/DHA improves the effectiveness of antidepressant drugs by helping the serotonin molecules fit better into the receptor sites on brain cell membranes.

In one study, sixty patients with a diagnosis of major depressive disorder were divided into three groups: those who received 1000 mg of EPA fish oil daily, those who received 20 mg of Prozac daily, and those who received a combination of the two.[21] Results showed that the combination of Prozac plus EPA was more effective than either of them alone. The results of those who received EPA alone compared with those who received Prozac alone showed that both were equally effective, but the fish oil takers suffered no side effects. Other studies showing clear benefits of omega-3 fish oil for depression and bipolar disorder were so convincing that the American Psychiatric Association now recommends a dosage greater than 1000 mg per day of EPA/DHA fish oil in addition to appropriate psychotropic drugs for treatment of mood disorders.

Mood Mellowers for Teens

I'm concerned that so many young people are taking prescription drugs for mood problems. Can fish oil help?

Yes. A study of seventy-six adolescents and young adults, ages 13–25 years, with early mood disorders given doses of 700 mg EPA and 480 mg DHA, compared with a placebo, showed fewer depressive symptoms and a slower progression of psychoses among those who took omega-3s. The scientific uncertainty that prescription antipsychotic drugs do any good, coupled with their particularly harmful effects in adolescents, is leading many doctors to reduce the use of these medicines in young people.[22]

Skills and Pills

I just don't like taking prescription medicines unless absolutely necessary. What else can I do to steady my mood?

Practice the skills-and-pills model of health care and self-care. Because the science that antidepressants offer real help is soft, and experience reveals that they can have serious side effects (e.g., mood flattening instead of mood mellowing, gastrointestinal disturbances, blood sugar instability, and excessive weight gain), the scientists I have consulted unanimously suggest, Try skills before pills:

- Get therapy, such as cognitive behavior therapy, which teaches you how to handle your moods.
- Move! Consistent, vigorous exercise is one of the healthiest mood mellowers. Studies show that in many patients with depression, daily vigorous exercise is as effective as, and safer than, prescription antidepressants.[23]
- Go fish! Studies show the dosage for beneficial results for mood disorders is 1000–6000 mg (1–6 grams) of EPA per day, with most studies getting positive results at 2000 mg (2 grams) of EPA per day. (For neurological disorders dosages, see pages 154–155.)

A therapeutic dose of omega-3s, unlike prescription antidepressants, follows the main mantra of medicine: first, do no harm. The science that omega-3s do no harm (and likely do good) for mood disorders is solid.

More Skills, Fewer Pills. Here's a depressing story with a happy ending. My wife, Martha, consulted her doctor about her menopausal symptoms of depression and was prescribed an SSRI antidepressant. Strike one! In my opinion, in most cases primary care doctors should not prescribe SSRIs. If needed, these medications should be prescribed by a psychiatrist, or by a psychopharmacologist, a physician who specializes in drug treatment of mood disorders.

After that, Martha's mood became flat: no joy, only sadness. She couldn't sleep. Back to her doctor, who added a sleeping pill to her drug regimen. Next, she became more anxious. Her doctor then referred her to a psychiatrist, who added a third drug to lower her anxiety. Martha got worse. No joy, no motivation, no libido. Strike two! Dubbed the "cocktail effect," this multiple-drug prescribing has a problem: Many of these drugs are tested and approved for single use only rather than in combination with other drugs.

Next, the psychiatrist concluded, "Perhaps you are suffering from side effects of one or more of these drugs. Let's try to wean you off one or two." Martha then got worse, prompting the doctor to conclude that she did, after all, need these drugs. Strike three! Most likely Martha's worsening symptoms were mainly due to the withdrawal effect: the brain habituates, getting so dependent upon prescription mood mellowers that it forgets how to make its own. I call this "the hole." The doctor is in a hole: Are the patient's problems the results of the drug or the disorder? The patient is in a hole, feeling helpless and hopeless. And family members are in a hole, understanding neither why the person they love is feeling so bad nor what they should do.

After six months of delving into the scientific literature during my crash course in psychopharmacology, I concluded that Martha was suffering more from the side effects of the drugs than from the disease. Along with 3000 mg of omega-3 EPA/DHA daily, what she needed was a "washout," a slow weaning off all drugs under expert professional supervision, and noting which symptoms got better and which got worse. It took a lot of personal work and consultation with a new psychiatrist, qualified in psychotherapy and medicine, to come out of this hole. Martha's solution over time was a combination of adjusting to the changes in her life through therapy, nutrition, exercise, and spiritual renewal, and her daily 3000 mg dose of omega-3s.

A LADYLIKE OMEGA-3 EFFECT

At the 2012 Global Organization for EPA and DHA (GOED) I invited a female speaker to join our all-male group of speakers at dinner, explaining, "Women add calmness to male conversation." Omega-3 scientist Dr. Michael Crawford quipped, "Like DHA calms the brain."

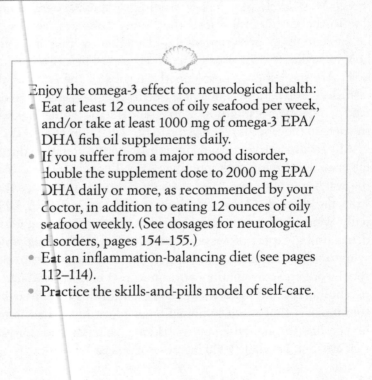

Enjoy the omega-3 effect for neurological health:
- Eat at least 12 ounces of oily seafood per week, and/or take at least 1000 mg of omega-3 EPA/DHA fish oil supplements daily.
- If you suffer from a major mood disorder, double the supplement dose to 2000 mg EPA/DHA daily or more, as recommended by your doctor, in addition to eating 12 ounces of oily seafood weekly. (See dosages for neurological disorders, pages 154–155.)
- Eat an inflammation-balancing diet (see pages 112–114).
- Practice the skills-and-pills model of self-care.

5

. . .

How Omega-3s Help Childhood Ds

At a recent school meeting with parents and teachers I presented some new and encouraging insights into treating ADHD/ADD and a lot of other Ds that affect children's ability to learn and behave, often resulting in Ds for grades. Approximately 10 percent of schoolchildren are now labeled with ADHD/ADD. And I'm concerned about these children getting too much of another D—drugs (prescription medicines). I assured my audience that there was a safer, better response than labeling and drugging. Of course, I realize many of these children are helped by *pills,* but I also want to give parents some additional *skills.*

I opened our discussion with a question: "Would a few of you parents tell me what your children had for breakfast this morning?"

There were various answers, from sweetened and colored cereals, to doughnuts, to no breakfast at all. Next, I asked, "How much fish do your children eat?" The general response was, "Not very much."

"How often do you see fish served in school lunches?" I asked the teachers.

"Seldom" was the answer.

When I asked how many parents understood how omega-3 foods improve kids' behavior and learning, only a few hands went up.

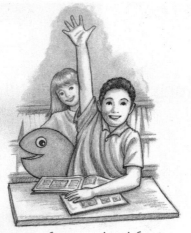

Seafood is school food.

I then stunned the audience with another D. "Many of these children don't have ADD. They have NDD, nutrition deficit disorder."

TO READ, WRITE, SPELL, AND BEHAVE BETTER, GO FISH!

I then showed the parents and teachers a visually striking example of a landmark study called the Oxford-Durham Study, done with a group of children in 2005.[1] This study set the bar for the use of omega-3s for children with behavioral or learning problems.

In 2005, British researchers at the University of Oxford studied 117 children, ages 5–12 years, who had what was called DCD (developmental coordination disorder), a catchall category that included behavioral and learning problems such as ADHD/ADD. Half the children were given an omega-3 supplement (558 mg EPA plus 174 mg DHA), and the other half took placebos. After three months the children taking omega-3s showed significant improvements in reading, spelling, and behavior. The children on placebos showed no improvement. Then the researchers put all the children on omega-3s for an additional three months, and those originally on placebos showed improvements similar to the original omega-3 takers.

The results of this study were so convincing that rumor has it that the children's teachers lobbied, although unsuccessfully, to be allowed to dispense omega-3 supplements to their students. The illustrations show an example of the remarkable improvement in the handwriting of an eight-year-old boy before (top) and after (bottom) he took omega-3 EPA/DHA supplements.

A Child's Handwriting Before
Omega-3 EPA/DHA Supplementation . . .

. . . and One Month After Supplementation:

In 2010, researchers at the University of Cincinnati studied thirty-three healthy boys, ages 8–10 years, and assigned them to three groups: one group got a placebo; the second group received 400 mg per day of DHA; and the third group received 1200 mg per day of DHA. The DHA levels in the red blood cells increased in the DHA-supplemented group by 47 percent and 70 percent, respectively, while the placebo group experienced an 11 percent drop in DHA levels. The scientists then performed fMRI brain scans during performance tests. The brain scans showed that both DHA-supplemented groups experienced significant activity increases in the prefontal cortex, the area of the brain associated with memory. The boys taking the higher dose of DHA showed better attention and speedier reaction time.[2]

He seems more content when he takes omega-3s.
— *Mother of a seven-year-old in our medical practice*

HOW OMEGA-3S HELP LEARNING AND BEHAVIOR

Chapter 4 explained how the omega-3 fats EPA and DHA make the brain tissue stronger and improve its functioning. Naturally, this omega-3 effect would be even more pronounced in the growing brains of children. Here's my take on why omega-3 deficiency contributes to childhood Ds, and why omega-3 supplements help avoid them. Omega-3 DHA is the top fat in the brain. It makes sense that the smarter the fats the child eats, the better the brain works. Remember, good science and common sense go together, and when they don't, suspect faulty science. If many of the childhood Ds are due to a deficiency or imbalance of neurohormones, such as serotonin and dopamine, and optimal nerve cell fluidity is necessary for these neurotransmitters to work, it makes sense to feed the brain more omega-3s. Eating more smart fats can produce a smarter and better-behaved brain. I believe that the rise in Ds at all ages parallels the oil change of the standard American diet (SAD). As kids began eating more factory-processed foods and oils and less fish oil, they got more Ds.

Serve Kids Real Foods. Real foods help the developing brain make real connections.

Oftentimes, rather than label children as having one of the Ds, I simply call them "quirky kids." Some children think, act, and learn differently because their brains are wired differently. They think outside the box, but given the right nutrition, supportive parenting, and a teaching style that matches the child's learning style, these children grow up to build better boxes. They can make this world a more interesting place. Yet the brains of these quirky children are more vulnerable to nutritional deficiencies, especially a deficiency of omega-3s. Consequently, they are more vulnerable to quirky moods and behaviors.

I believe that the brains of growing children need sufficient dietary omega-3s and a ratio of about 2:1 to 3:1 of omega 6s to omega-3s. How do we know that? We study Mother Nature, who

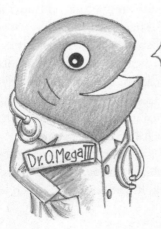

For better-behaved brains, give your child an oil change.

does not make nutritional mistakes nor continually change her mind about nutritional advice. Mother's milk averages a ratio of 2:1 to 3:1 omega 6s to omega-3s. The ratio of these fats in wild meats and wild fish is around 2:1, yet the ratio in the SAD is 10:1. Just serve real food and make sure some of it comes from the sea. (See recommended dosages of seafood and fish oil supplements, Chapter 11.)

FISH STORIES OF SCHOOL SUCCESS

Here are some testimonies from the Sears Pediatrics and Family Medicine practice.

A Mother's Testimony after Giving Her Child an Oil Change

"Because of my adopted son's prenatal exposure to heroin, methadone, and we're not sure what else, he was diagnosed with sensory integration syndrome. Simply stated, the neurons in his brain and body don't communicate properly. His difficulties started in first grade. He had trouble concentrating, poor writing skills and low grades at school. He lied and was angry and destructive. Any normal task would take numerous reminders.

"I was told repeatedly by teachers, special education assessors, and all the other academic specialists that the only course of action was to put him on ADHD medication. Just as I was about to give up and put him on the medication, I consulted Dr. Sears, who prescribed 1000 mg of omega-3 EPA/DHA fish oil daily, in addition to serving him salmon twice a week. Quite honestly, I thought it a bit odd, but I started his fish oil the next day.

"Within two to three days he was calmer, not 'zoned out' or 'spacey,' just relaxed. He was still sharp, funny, and a bit sassy, but not disrespectful. Within a week, life at home was much less stressful, and he was getting along better with everyone. There was laughter in my house again. Within two weeks his schoolwork improved, and homework is not the ordeal it once was. His comprehension skills were above grade level and his writing was legible. We had spent thousands of dollars on tutoring, therapies, and various programs designed for learning-disabled children. Now he is at the top of his class.

"This has been nothing short of our own personal miracle. You have given me my son back! Thank you, Dr. Sears!"

A Success Story of a Teacher's Child

"Because I am a teacher, I knew Abby had ADD. Needless to say, I was concerned and realized Abby's inability to focus may interfere with finishing first grade. She couldn't remember sight words or homework assignments, and we visited lost-and-found daily to pick up lunch boxes or jackets that she would leave around the school.

"I called my mom because I knew she would understand the situation, as she was also a schoolteacher, though retired. After hearing the story, she said, 'I just returned from a nutrition talk by Dr. Bill Sears. Tracee, you need to get Abby on omega-3s because the neurotransmitters in her brain need them for clear thinking. Your body does not make enough omega-3s, you need to eat foods with them. If she won't eat fish, give her fish oil.'

"I ordered fish oil capsules and began giving them to her. Before a week was over, I received a note from her teacher asking me what I had done because Abby was focused. She was answering questions for the first time. I continue to give Abby omega-3s. She is delighted that she is really able to learn. She is one of the best students in her class. I cringe to think that she might have repeated first grade unnecessarily.

"P.S. This big change in Abby inspired me to find out if

students in my fifth-grade class took omega-3 fish oils. I was not surprised to find out that all my top students took them."

OMEGA-3 QUESTIONS YOU MAY HAVE

Epidemic of Ds

Why in recent years are we seeing such a strong epidemic of Ds?

Unfortunately, no one knows the complete answer. I believe some children are born with a genetic vulnerability, a sort of switch in their genes that when turned on produces a D. These vulnerable kids might be repeatedly exposed to environmental toxins and artificial chemicals in foods, which switches on their D gene.

Here's another theory popular among omega-3 researchers. They believe that during pregnancy and lactation most expectant mothers now take omega-3s; infant formulas are fortified with omega-3s; and breast milk has omega-3s in it, so most babies get some omega-3s. Then something happens. During infancy, toddlerhood and the preschool years, the stages of most rapid brain growth, kids often no longer eat enough omega-3s. Omega-3 deficiencies keep the brain from making the right connections. If this window of brain growth opportunity is missed, by the time the child gets to school, the brain is quirky, and the child could be labeled with a D. Nutritional studies revealed that only 22 percent of children, ages 4–8 years, ate adequate omega-3 EPA/DHA daily.[3]

Autism

I have a son with autism. Could omega-3s help him?[4]

Children with autism should be given at least 1000 mg per day of fish oil either in supplements or seafood. While studies of the omega-3 effect in children with autism are few, many other studies support the beneficial effects of omega-3 supplements in children with behavior and learning problems, both of which occur in children with autism. For more about the value of omega-3s and other supplements that can help kids with autism, read *The Autism Book,* by Robert Sears, MD (Little, Brown, 2010).

SCIENCE SAYS: OMEGA-3 EPA/DHA IS A SMART FOOD FOR SCHOOLKIDS

- Children with low blood levels of omega-3s are more likely to suffer from the Ds, such as ADHD, OCD (obsessive compulsive disorder), and CDs (conduct disorders).
- Children with ADHD were found to have low blood levels of the most brainy omega-3, DHA.
- In cultures where people eat more omega-3s, for example, in Asian and some Mediterranean cultures, there is a much lower incidence of nearly all the Ds.
- In schoolchildren taking fish oil supplements, those with the highest blood levels of omega-3s achieved better test performance and better attention than others.[5]
- Many studies show that omega-3 supplementation improved ADHD symptoms, with no side effects.[6]
- The neurosurgeon Dr. Russell Blaylock reported that a study of boys, ages 6–12 years, found that those with the lowest levels of omega-3s demonstrated more episodes of violent and angry behavior and problems with impulse control than others.[7] In another study, students who took fish oil supplements (1500–1800 mg) showed less aggressive behavior than others in times of mental stress.[8] Other studies have shown that diets deficient in omega-3s may trigger violent behavior.
- Another D that may be helped by eating more omega-3 EPA/DHA is dyslexia. A study of twenty Swedish children with dyslexia showed they improved in reading speed by 60 percent after taking supplements with fish oil.[9]

Teaching Kids about Omega-3s

I'd like to teach my class about the health benefits of omega-3s. Any tips?

Since the brain is the organ most affected, for better or worse, by nutrition, and omega-3s are one of the top brain nutrients, it's a perfect fit. More about these supernutrients should be taught in schools. Here are some suggestions, most of which I have personally tried, and they work.

- *Play "Simon Says."* Remember the KISMIF teaching principle: keep it simple, make it fun. If your child knows and likes the game "Simon Says," play "Salmon Says" as you go through the head-to-toe health benefits of omega-3s: "Salmon says I make brains smarter"; "Salmon says I help eyes see better"; "Salmon says I help your heart beat stronger so you can play sports better"; "Salmon says I help you have smoother, softer skin"; "Salmon says I'm a muscle food. I help you be stronger."

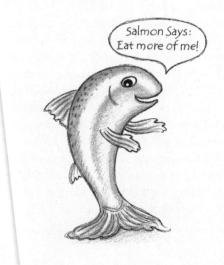

- *Make it relevant.* Kids are looks- and performance-oriented, not health nuts—yet. Since "healthy" may be perceived as icky by some children, present seafood as "soccer food," "football food," "get-better-grades food," "pretty skin food." You could even ask your class, "Who would like to make higher grades?" When they raise their hands, say "Go fish!" "Who would like to have more energy, play sports better, and not get sick as often?" As they raise their hands, say "Go fish!"
- *Make it memorable.* If some children in the class want you to go deeper to explain why seafood is good for them, make omegas memorable for them. Say, "Inside fish or fish oil capsules are nutrients called omega-3s. Let's call them megs. They are sort of like the bricks and wood when you build a building. That's why we call megs 'grow foods.' They make every organ of your body grow better. The two main megs that are your grow foods are called EPA and DHA." Have the children try to pronounce eicosapentaenoic acid and docosahexaenoic acid. Trying to say these tongue-twisting words will help them remember the words, or at least that omega-3s are important.

Since children are computer-oriented, say, "Look at that computer screen. It says 'Intel Inside.' That Intel is like the brain of your computer. Megs are to your brain and body what the 'Intel Inside' is to your computer. So picture your brain saying: 'Megs inside.' "

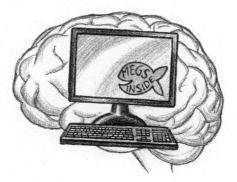

- *Explain how megs make you healthier.* Kids love the sticky stuff analogy of illness. Try: "When people get sick, tired, and have sore joints, they get sticky stuff on their tissues, mainly their blood vessels. Now let me show you what happens when you get sticky stuff inside your blood vessels. And, you know, doctors have discovered sticky stuff on the lining of blood vessels in kids as young as five years old. You need healthy blood vessels to supply all the nourishment and the energy to your muscles that help you run and dance, and your brain helps you think and play video games and outwit the computer. When you put too much sticky stuff in your mouth, year after year, that sticky stuff gradually builds up, sort of like plaque on your teeth. Remember how the dentist has to scrape all that sticky stuff off your teeth? The same thing happens in your blood vessels. Over time it gradually builds up until your muscles and brain and all your other organs don't get enough nourishment through your blood, and that's what makes you sick and weak. It also makes your skin look old. Your brain can't think as fast on the video games. You can't run as fast or play soccer as well." (See the illustration on page 61 showing buildup of plaque in arteries from age 10 to age 50.)
- *Teach traffic-light eating.* Make a list of green-light foods, which you can present as "enjoy anytime, eat as much as you want." Yellow-light foods are treats: "enjoy, but not too much." Too much and you get sticky stuff in your tissues. Red-light foods are "stop—make a better choice." Those are sticky foods that cause sticky stuff to build up in your blood vessels. (See the traffic-light table of seafoods, pages 186–187, and *The Healthiest Kids in the Neighborhood* (Little, Brown, 2006) for a list of traffic-light foods.)
- *Give them homework.* Give your children a memorable game to play at home: "Tonight go into your pantry and

fridge and play 'I spy with my little eyes.' Every food that you see that has a bad word on the label, a red-light food (the bad words are *high fructose corn syrup, hydrogenated,* and a # color symbol, such as *red #40*), put it in a box. When you present the box to your daddy, he then owes you a quarter for every red-light food you find."

• *Take kids shopping.* Use the supermarket as a giant nutritional classroom. Compare the steak and seafood sections: "That piece of steak is a muscle from an animal that sat around and ate junk food all day. That salmon fillet is from a fish that jumped out of the water, swam upstream, ate good food, and exercised much of the day. Do you want your muscles to be weak and flabby like the steak or strong like the salmon?" Children get it.

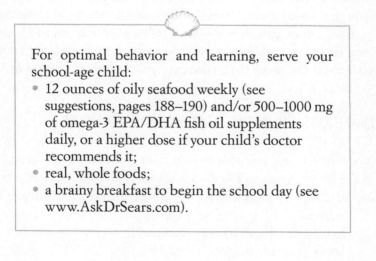

For optimal behavior and learning, serve your school-age child:
• 12 ounces of oily seafood weekly (see suggestions, pages 188–190) and/or 500–1000 mg of omega-3 EPA/DHA fish oil supplements daily, or a higher dose if your child's doctor recommends it;
• real, whole foods;
• a brainy breakfast to begin the school day (see www.AskDrSears.com).

6

Enjoy the Omega-3 Effect during Pregnancy and Your Child's Infancy

Expectant and new mothers, you'll be happy to know that one simple oil change can help you enjoy a healthier pregnancy and have a smarter baby. While eating more omega-3s is health-building for all ages, there is a stage of life when the omega-3 effect may have the most profound influence: during pregnancy and your child's infancy.[1] Here's how to give your baby a smart start.

OMEGA-3S PROMOTE HEALTHY PREGNANCIES

You'll be amazed how this one nutrient contributes so much to a healthier pregnancy. Here's a summary of what science says. Mothers who ate more omega-3s during their pregnancy enjoyed:

- lower risk of high blood pressure;[2]
- lower risk of high blood sugar;[3]
- slightly lower risk of delivering a premature infant or a baby with less than optimal birth weight;[4]
- less depression before and after delivery;[5]

- babies who have better visual acuity, especially if premature;[6]
- infants who have fewer allergies, such as asthma and eczema;[7]
- babies who tend to sleep better;[8]
- children who have a higher IQ.[9]

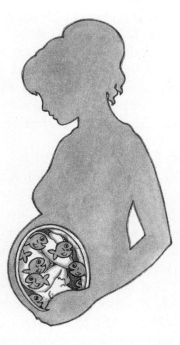

Besides the research showing that pregnant mothers who eat sufficient omega-3s lower their risk of medical problems, there is a piece of research that has gotten mixed reviews among pregnant mothers. Researchers found that mothers who take omega-3 supplements during pregnancy have an increase in the duration of their pregnancy by three to six days and reduce the risk of delivering a premature baby. Scientists believe that is because omega-3s help regulate prostaglandins, the chemical messengers that initiate uterine contractions.[10] This may not be welcome news to those of you who can't wait for your delivery day, but a few more days in your womb greatly increase the chance of your baby's being born with healthier lungs and fewer problems associated with prematurity. Anything you can do to increase maturity is good for your baby.

Preterm infants are at higher risk for omega-3 deficiency and are therefore more likely to benefit from omega-3 supplements than term infants for two reasons. First, preterm babies have less body fat and therefore less of a storage bank for omega-3s. Second, they have had less time to store omega-3s in their tissues. So it's wise to plan ahead by loading baby up with omega-3s early in the pregnancy in case he or she is born prematurely.

OMEGA-3S MAKE NEW MOMS HAPPIER

What's good for baby is good for mom. Not only does eating extra omega-3s by women during pregnancy result in smarter and healthier babies; new research suggests it may help mothers be happier during pregnancy and after birth.

It's exhausting being a mother. With all the change of routine and lack of sleep, it's no wonder moms get worn out and feeling low. Though the science is still in its infancy, research suggests that the more omega-3s mothers eat during pregnancy and after birth, the less likely they are to suffer postpartum depression. Here's my theory on why.

Research links depression with low omega-3 blood levels. Studies show that maternal blood levels of omega-3s decline after delivery. After birth it takes several months for mothers' omega-3 blood level values to return to normal. This stands to reason, since the baby, a little nutritional parasite, gets first dibs on available nutrition, sometimes at the expense of the mother's health.

The baby diverts the omega-3s it needs from the mother's blood during pregnancy and breast-feeding. Baby literally sucks the omega-3s out of mom, leaving her with an omega-3 deficiency. Mother should take in enough omega-3s for both herself and her baby.

The field of psychoneuroendocrinology reveals another reason pregnant mothers should eat more omega-3s. During the last trimester, a pregnant woman's immune system perks up to protect both mother and baby from infection and to prepare the mother's body for birth. These high levels of proinflammatory and protective biochemicals, called cytokines, need to be balanced by high levels of omega-3s (see inflammatory balance, page 114). If the levels of cytokines get too high, this can lead to abnormalities in sleep, energy, and moods.[11] These new insights put postpartum depression within the spectrum of inflammation disorders, or -*itis* illnesses. The potent anti-inflammatory effect of omega-3s puts a bit of a brake on the mother's hyped-up immune system and helps mellow her moods.

OMEGA-3S MAKE BABY BRAINS BRIGHTER

A baby's brain grows most rapidly in the third trimester of pregnancy through the first two years of life. Research reveals that a baby's brain growing in the womb extracts the most DHA from mother's blood during the last three months of her pregnancy. The amount of brain DHA builds up from about 22 weeks' gestation to 2 years of age, the period of most rapid brain growth. Since the brain is 60 percent fat and omega-3 DHA is a top fat in the brain, it makes sense to feed your child more omega-3s during and after your pregnancy.

Infancy and toddlerhood are critical windows of brain development during which nerves must go through two growth features:

myelination and nerve connections, both of which depend on adequate omega-3s in the baby's diet. If these trillions of nerves are not both myelinated and connected during this window of rapid brain development, they are pruned, meaning the body treats them like weeds or useless plants that must be pulled out or cut. (See myelination, pages 65–66.)

A study of forty-eight hundred children compared a group whose mothers had taken fish oil supplements during pregnancy to a control group whose mothers had received a placebo, and found higher scores on intelligence tests in the supplements group children at age 4. The mothers took fish oil supplements containing 2000 mg per day of omega-3s from 18 weeks' gestation until their infants were 3 months old.[12]

The more myelination and connections a child's brain goes through in its first five years, the smarter the brain develops.

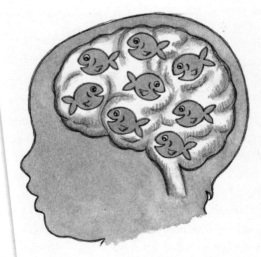

"My brain is going through a
growth spurt."

Omega-3s provide the nutrients that enable this to happen. If babies' brains could talk, they would say, "I'm going through a growth spurt, feed me smart foods so I can think faster, and help me make the right connections." That's why some pediatricians call omega-3s grow foods.

A single nerve fiber, or neuron, in the brain may make as many as twenty thousand connections with other nerve fibers during its life. If you were a developing brain and your intelligence depended on the connections you made with other nerve fibers, wouldn't that be where you would concentrate the smart fats? That's exactly what the brain does. These connections, called synapses, have a higher concentration of DHA than nearly any other tissue in the body. The more connections, the smarter the brain.

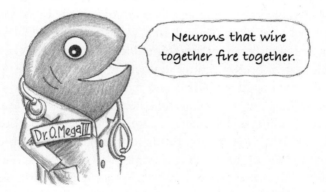

Neurons that wire together fire together.

Dr. O. Mega III

Just in case you aren't convinced, here's a clincher. If I were to ask, "What's the most exhausting part of being a new mother?" a chorus of tired moms would shout, "Sleep! Lack of sleep!" A study showed that mothers who had high levels of omega-3s in their blood during pregnancy had babies who enjoyed more mature sleep patterns.[13]

Before you all rush out to buy a bottle of fish oil or go to your nearest seafood market, there is a lot more you need to know. So let's go fishing for more information.

OMEGA-3S MAKE "SMART" BREAST MILK

Science confirms what breast-feeding moms intuitively suspect: breast-fed babies are smarter and healthier. When researchers studied a group of children breast-fed as infants, they found that the duration of breast-feeding correlated positively with the child's IQ at 6½ years of age.[14]

Yet research reveals that the content of DHA in the breast milk of North American mothers tends to be lower than in many other cultures where mothers eat more seafood.[15]

Mothers who eat the standard American diet make milk that is considerably lower in omega-3s than milk made by women in cultures who eat more seafood. In a 2006 study of the DHA content of breast milk of mothers from nine countries, DHA content was highest in breast-feeding mothers in Japan and the Arctic cultures, and lowest in Canada and the United States.[16]

Researchers put these clues together. Studies showed that the brain tissue of breast-fed infants contained higher proportions of DHA than the brains of formula-fed babies.[17] Could the IQ increase be due to the rich level of omega-3 EPA/DHA in mother's milk? The same research showed that breast-feeding mothers who took omega-3 supplements had a higher content of EPA/DHA in their breast milk.

In the United States the omega-6 (linoleic acid) content in breast milk increased from 6–7 percent of total fatty acids in 1945 to 15–16 percent in 1995, reflecting a steady increase in omega-6s in mothers' diets. Some researchers are concerned that this increase in omega-6s may weaken the omega-3 effect of breast milk. (See omega balance, page 29.)

Putting all this together, the conclusion of medical experts was that mothers should continue their prenatal omega-3 supplements while breast-feeding. As a bit of encouragement for mothers who are tempted to wean early, imagine that every time you breast-feed your baby, you are giving your baby a dose of "smart milk."

COMMON QUESTIONS PREGNANT MOTHERS HAVE

Fertility Fertilizer

Can omega-3s affect sperm count?

Omega-3s are good for fertility. It seems that all things that swim need omega-3s.

A study of men attending a fertility clinic found that a higher intake of omega-3s was related to higher-quality, better-formed sperm.[18] And although what happens to mice doesn't always happen to men, a 2011 study showed that feeding DHA restored fertility in mice.[19] The seminiferous tubules, the tissue in the testes where sperm grows, are loaded with omega-3s. So, guys, go fish!

Omega Prenatal Dosage

How much omega-3 should I take during pregnancy and breast-feeding?

Here's what I recommend in our medical practice, and why. While pregnant and breast-feeding, eat 12 ounces of safe seafood per week (see Appendixes B–C for safe seafood selections), and take 500 mg of omega-3 EPA/DHA supplements daily. This will give you about 1000 mg of omega-3s daily. Or, if you can't stomach seafood, take 1000 mg of omega-3 EPA/DHA from fish oil supplements daily. A dose of 500 mg daily is the standard figure for all adults. Since the baby's rapidly growing body and brain need extra nutrients, especially omega-3s, it makes sense for a pregnant mother to eat more omega-3s than a nonpregnant person. Since you may have special nutritional needs, always check the dosages of all supplements with your health care provider.

Here's how I arrived at the 1000 mg daily dose. Omega-3 authorities agree that there are no safety issues with 1000 mg of omega-3s per day for any adult, including mothers during pregnancy and lactation. The recommendations of the most trusted authorities, such as the International Society for the Study of Fatty Acids and Lipids and the National Institutes of Health, is 500 mg per day as "the minimum preventive medicine requirement for all adults." If 500 mg is the recommendation for all adults, and it goes up to 4000 mg per day for adults with cardiovascular and neurological problems, then certainly a pregnant woman must need more than 500 mg.

So let's see whose tissues need those extra omega-3s. First, the growing baby. The baby's brain is growing faster than at any other time during life, and omega-3s are one of the prime essential fats for brain growth. Various estimates are about 70 mg DHA per day to 25 mg per pound, especially during the brain growth spurt in the third trimester.[20] So let's say about 200 mg per day for the baby, to be on the safe side.

Then we have mother's blood volume increasing around 40 percent to an extra couple of quarts. Red blood cell membranes are rich in omega-3s. While exact figures are hard to come by, for safety's sake let's add another 100 mg. Then we have a lot of extra uterine muscle, placenta, and breast-milk-producing tissue, so add another 200 mg for the mother's body. The science is still uncertain and we're left with intelligent estimates. That gives a minimum of 1000 mg (1 gram) per day of combined DHA and EPA (at least 500 mg per day should be DHA) for the health of mother and baby.

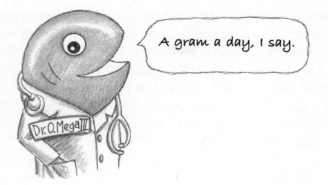

Good Fats vs. Bad Fats; Good Fish vs. Bad Fish

In addition to eating more good fats while I'm pregnant, are there bad fats I shouldn't eat?

Yes. While inside your womb, your baby's growing brain uses 70 percent of all the food energy that goes through your placenta. Remember, smart fats make the proper-fitting locks for nerve keys to fit into and grow more connections. When dumb fats (hydrogenated oils) cross the placenta, they clog the locks so the keys don't fit. Hydrogenated oils, also called trans fats, can block the enzymes needed to manufacture DHA from ALA. While scientists aren't sure how much of the hydrogenated oils that mom eats crosses the placenta to the baby, don't take a chance. Avoid dumb fats, and eat smart fats.

Omega-3 Dosage for Babies

How much omega-3 should I give my baby each day?

Since there is no official government Recommended Daily Intake (RDI) for omega-3s, I'm frequently asked how much daily omega-3 DHA infants should eat. (Since most of the studies focus on DHA, not EPA, I discuss only DHA here.) I reviewed what science says, consulted experts, and did the math. The average breast-fed-only infant at about 6 months of age would get about 760 ml (27 ounces) of breast milk daily. (Babies average 2–2.5 ounces per pound per day in their first 6 months.) Assuming an average fat concentration of 40 grams/liter, a mother with optimal daily DHA consumption would yield about 300 mg DHA per day to her baby.[21] Based on this reasoning, I advise mothers to be sure their infants get about 300 mg DHA per day from breast milk, DHA-fortified infant formula, omega-3 DHA supplements, or seafood. (See Chapter 11 for more dosage information.)

Vegetarian Diet

Is my vegetarian diet okay for my baby?

Be prudent while you're pregnant. Take 1000 mg per day of omega-3 supplements. Some studies show that DHA levels are low in vegetarians. DHA levels are typically lower in the blood of infants born to vegetarian mothers, and DHA blood levels of breast-fed infants of vegetarian mothers are only about one-third the level of nonvegetarians. Vegans (no animal products or seafood) must supplement their otherwise healthy diet with many nutrients, especially omega-3s. (See Chapter 11 for more dosage information.)

Feeding Fish to Babies

How early should I begin feeding seafood to our baby?

Alaskan natives feed their infants fish eggs, called salmon roe (a rich source of omega-3s), at about 8 months of age. At the 2012 ISSFAL meeting I overheard a top omega-3 researcher saying, "We give our nine-month-old salmon roe." In our medical practice I advise patients to introduce wild salmon into the baby's diet at about 8–9 months of age. Begin with a fingertipful of soft baked meat. Increase the amount and preparations as the baby's ability to chew textures increases.

The magic words of infant feeding are "shape young tastes." Called metabolic programming by nutrition researchers, it's like the gut brain gets programmed to crave what is best for the body. I've noticed that infants who eat seafood early are more likely to like seafood later.

Here's a fish story from our daughter Hayden:

> I started giving all three of my children wild salmon at age 8 or 9 months. I wanted to start early so that they would get used to fish and consider it a staple food. I usually poached or baked it with lemon juice and fed it to them from my plate. At first I just gave them little bits mashed between my fingers. As they got older, I would give them more and more. Sharing it from my plate made it something special. When my toddlers went through stages where they did not want salmon, I would mash it up in their sweet potatoes or layer it with shredded cheese in quesadillas until they were happy to eat chunks of it again.

(See Chapter 12 on serving fish to kids.)

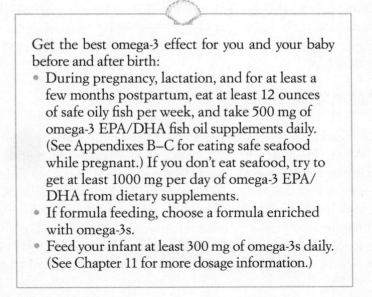

Get the best omega-3 effect for you and your baby before and after birth:
- During pregnancy, lactation, and for at least a few months postpartum, eat at least 12 ounces of safe oily fish per week, and take 500 mg of omega-3 EPA/DHA fish oil supplements daily. (See Appendixes B–C for eating safe seafood while pregnant.) If you don't eat seafood, try to get at least 1000 mg per day of omega-3 EPA/ DHA from dietary supplements.
- If formula feeding, choose a formula enriched with omega-3s.
- Feed your infant at least 300 mg of omega-3s daily. (See Chapter 11 for more dosage information.)

7

. . .

How Omega-3s Help -*itis* Illnesses

Doctors spend much of their time treating patients suffering from -*itis* illnesses: arthritis, bronchitis (asthma), colitis (inflammatory bowel disease), and dermatitis (eczema), and another -*itis* that I call cognitivitis, better known as Alzheimer's disease. Pharmaceutical companies cater to these patients, who annually spend over $20 billion on anti-inflammatory drugs. Many people with stiff, achy, itchy, and bloated bodies are starting to think there must be a safer way to heal their hurts. There is: Go fish!

ARE YOU AN IBOD?

One day I was counseling a whole family with a variety of -*itis* illnesses. I opened with, "Welcome, iBods!" This statement startled them. They hadn't heard the term *iBod* before. They didn't know what it meant, but they certainly didn't want to be iBods.

An iBod is what I call a body riddled with inflammation. Inflammation means your immune system is on fire and out of control. If you are an iBod, you take pills for your ills, yet you are scared by the side effects of these medications. Many of these medicines have had bad press lately. The good news is that there is a "medicine" that helps put out the fire inside your body. This medicine

- is biochemically an anti-inflammatory;
- occurs in nature, so it is truly natural;
- has no harmful side effects;
- does not need a prescription;
- is relatively inexpensive.

Of course, you know by now that I'm talking about the omega-3s.

THE CONCEPT OF INFLAMMATORY BALANCE

Your immune system is genetically programmed to search out foreign invaders (germs) and destroy them before they can damage your tissues. Inside your body you have two armies. One group, let's call it "the fighters," kills invading enemy germs. This battle causes inflammation. Biochemically, the fighters are known as *proinflammatories*. The other group, let's call it "the healers," cleans up after the battle. The healers balance wear and tear with repair. These healing biochemicals are called *anti-inflammatories*. These armies are in *inflammatory balance* when the wear and tear of the body's biochemical battle is healed by just the right amount of repair.

If the wear and tear of the battle—inflammation—overwhelms the body's ability to repair its tissues, leaving rough, inflamed surfaces, those tissues have an *-itis,* for example, inflamed joint surfaces (arthritis) or inflamed airways (bronchitis). The worst-case scenario of immune system trouble happens when the fighters get confused and attack the body's own tissues when germs aren't even there. When the body attacks itself, it's called having an *autoimmune* disease.

When you do too much chemical abuse (e.g., eat junk food) and physical abuse (e.g., sit too much) to your body, the foreign food chemicals that you eat (e.g., factory-made oils, chemical food additives) infiltrate your tissues. After this sticky stuff worms its way into healthy tissues, the tissues change their chemistry. The fighters in your immune system then wrongly conclude that these tissues—usually those that line joints, airways, intestines, and blood vessels—are foreign and don't belong there. So they attack them, causing inflammation. If you don't eat enough inflammation-balancing chemicals like omega-3s and antioxidants, tissue damage—*-itis*—results. The soreness you feel is the result of that losing battle being fought inside you.

OMEGA-3S ARE NATURAL ANTI-INFLAMMATORIES

Most people don't eat enough omega-3 fats. That's one reason they're iBods. Controlling inflammation is becoming the focus for keeping the body healthy at all ages. Inflammation simply means excessive wear and tear, or "rough edges," all over the body. The causes of chronic inflammation are many and complicated, but one thing you can do to help keep it in check is to eat more omega-3s. Omega-3s swim to all the cells of the body, injecting them with EPA and DHA to prime the immune system to help reduce inflammation. Omega-3 EPA/DHA prevents excessive inflammation by inhibiting overproduction of harmful inflamers (called inflammatory eicosanoids) and releasing healing biochemicals, such as resolvins and protectins. Omega-3 EPA is especially good at taming those inflamers.

Both doctors and patients continue to search for arthritis pain relievers that are safer than prescription drugs. They may have found one. In one study, doctors specializing in arthritis-induced back pain prescribed between 1200 and 2400 mg of fish oil per day to their patients. Of 125 patients taking fish oil for an average of seventy-five days, 60 percent reported improvement, and 59 percent were able to quit taking their prescription NSAID (*non*steroidal *a*nti-*in*flammatory *d*rug) medication.[1]

Some doctors recommend that you eat less omega-6 oil and more omega-3 oil. (See omega balance, page 29.) If you're like most iBods, eating ten times more omega-6 oil than omega-3 EPA/DHA oil, try changing your dietary ratio of omega-6s to omega-3s to 3:1. Omega-3s are the smooth operators that prevent

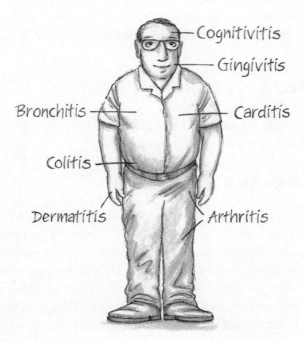

Don't be an iBod. Change your oils.

Cognitivitis
Gingivitis
Bronchitis
Carditis
Colitis
Dermatitis
Arthritis

excessive wear and tear and exaggerated repair. Their cousins, the omega-6s (vegetable oils, including soybean and corn oil, most salad dressings, and fried foods), are proinflammatory. When ingested in excess, they overstimulate the immune system, causing faulty repair. Dr. William Harris, a leading omega-3 scientist, emphasizes that you won't effectively tame inflammation just by eating less omega-6 oil. You must also eat more omega-3 EPA/DHA fish oil. Normally, when the omega-3s and the omega-6s peacefully coexist, the body is in inflammatory balance. When the omega-3s are insufficient to counteract the omega-6s, the body gets out of balance and becomes an iBod.

I prefer the term *inflammation-balancing* instead of *anti-inflammatory,* which is sort of like *anti-aging.* When you don't age, you don't live. Wellness is a body with inflammatory balance, and illness is a body with inflammatory imbalance. One way to help balance the fighters and healers in your immune system is to feed them the foods that fit their needs.

HOW OMEGA-3S BALANCE INFLAMMATION

Let's go on a health trip through your body to see how the omega-3 effect heals common *-itis* illnesses.

Omega-3s Are Blood Vessel Protectors

When your arteries get inflamed, the arterial lining gets sticky like Velcro instead of being smooth and nonsticky like silk. The body eventually perceives that the arteries are like a road in need of repair and sends out its repair crew to fix it. Yet sometimes the patching that the repair crew does (inflammation) slows traffic (blood flow), and this can lead to traffic jams (clotting). Omega-3s act as anti-inflammatories and anticoagulants that reduce clotting and damage to arterial walls. Omega-3s feed the maintenance crew so the workers can keep the surface of the road smooth and keep the traffic moving. These omega-3 EPA/DHA fats act in much the same way as aspirin and some of the prescription anticoagulant and anti-inflammatory drugs do, but they're much safer.

Omega-3s Tame Inflamed Tissues

Omega-3s reduce wear and tear in all tissues in the body, especially the joints. Most joints need oiling. Omega-3s are the best oil for sore joints. When any surface rubs against another surface, as the knee joint does when you walk, or as the blood flows against the artery walls when you run, you need the omega-3 effect to protect and keep tissues smooth.

Omega-3s are also good for the gut. They help tame inflammatory bowel disease, such as Crohn's disease. Omega-3s also help you breathe better. And these oils may help some kids and adults with allergies or allergic bronchitis, asthma. Omega-3s, especially EPA, work in a way similar to prescription and over-the-counter anti-inflammatory medicines but without their gastrointestinal side effects.

Omega-3s Help Prevent Inflammation in Cell Membranes

Remember, your body is only as healthy as each cell. The cell membrane is where omega-3s prevent inflammatory mischief. Inside the cell membrane are enzymes called COX. In an attempt to protect the membrane and the vital nutrients inside each cell, the COX enzymes inside the membrane biochemically convert the omega-3 EPA/DHA into potent anti-inflammatories to protect the cell from excess inflammatories, or wear and tear chemicals, called cytokines.

Within the cell membrane reside the omega-3s' cousins, omega-6s, namely, arachidonic acid, the excess of which can be proinflammatory. As long as these two omegas are balanced, the cell protects itself with balanced inflammation: kill foreign germs but not healthy cells. But when you eat a big burger and oily fries, a sugary drink, and a sticky dessert — lots of sticky fats and few omega-3s — the blood and all cell membranes are flooded with omega-6s. These excess omega-6s steal all the COX enzymes for their own use, so there are not enough left over to utilize the omega-3s. Then you've eaten your way into inflammatory imbalance: excess omega-6s (proinflammatory) and insufficient omega-3s (anti-inflammatory). You become a hurting iBod.

Here's what causes iBods to hurt, as with sore joints. The excess omega-6s are metabolized by the COX enzymes into chemicals called leukotrienes and eicosanoids. While these sound like the names of aliens from outer space, they are chemicals that build up in lining tissues, such as bronchi, blood vessels, joints, and intestines. They cause pain and swelling of these tissues. Over time these tissues become permanently damaged. How many of your friends go to a surgeon for hip or knee replacements?

Omega-3s Help Young iBods

Think -*itis* illnesses only happen to older folks? Think again. The way children eat today predisposes them to many illnesses: they are pre-diabetic, pre–cardiovascular disease, pre-arthritic, and pre- all those adult illnesses. Omega-3s help keep that from happening and can often reverse it once it starts so that kids are less likely to get all these diseases. These medical problems used to be called adult onset diseases. But now, because children are getting high blood pressure, high blood cholesterol, and high blood sugar, the term *adult onset* is no longer used in medical textbooks.

Omega-3s also help baby iBods. A fish oil supplementation

study of sixty-four healthy Danish infants who received formula with or without fish oil showed that the supplemented infants had higher omega-3 content in their red blood cell membranes in addition to fewer inflammatory markers,[2] meaning fewer circulating proinflammatory chemicals that lead to iBods. The trigger for this study was the observation that the immune system matures faster in breast-fed babies than in formula-fed infants. Grandmothers seemed to know this when giving infants and young children that daily distasteful spoonful of cod-liver oil, which was rich in omega-3s and other oils as well as vitamins A and D. Modern researchers later confirmed that, in this respect, grandma knew best.

Omega-3s Help Colitis

Colitis, or inflammatory bowel disease, can be helped by increased omega-3 intake.[3] Omega-3s are incorporated into the gut mucosa, intestinal lining cells, which may result in anti-inflammatory effects by decreasing inflammatory substances in bowel tissue.

Omega-3s Help You Breathe Easier

A study from Harvard University and Health Association Canada showed that teens who ate more omega-3s along with their fruits and vegetables had fewer symptoms of asthma and chronic bronchitis.[4] This stands to reason, since asthma is mainly bronchospasm due to excessive inflammation, and fruits, vegetables, and seafood are anti-inflammatory. What about exercise-induced asthma? Study results have been conflicting, so researchers generally agree that no definite conclusion can yet be drawn regarding the efficacy of omega-3 supplementation as a treatment for asthma in children and adults. Here's my take. Asthma is caused by inflammation. Omega-3s are anti-inflammatories. Go fish!

Omega-3s Can Help Diabetes

New insights reveal that often diabetes may be another -*itis* illness. In fact, a daily dose of fish oil and a fillet of salmon two or three times a week is the first prescription I write for my patients who already have diabetes or who want to lower the risk of getting it. If your family tree has a genetic tendency toward diabetes, the earlier you start your omega-3 preventive medicine, the better. The twelve-year Diabetes Autoimmunity Study in the Young (DAISY) studied 1,770 children who were genetically at high risk for developing type 1 diabetes. It found that kids who had the highest level of omega-3s in their red blood cell membranes were ultimately the least likely to develop type 1 diabetes.[5]

Omega-3s can also help the neuropathy (nerve damage) associated with diabetes. This makes sense, since the nerves are damaged by inflammation and myelin degeneration, and omega-3s are anti-inflammatories and myelin makers. Diabetics also tend to suffer from blood vessel stiffening and narrowing, or endothelium dysfunction. While omega-3s don't directly lower blood sugar and may not directly improve insulin sensitivity, they do help reduce the complications of diabetes, especially cardiovascular disease, stroke, high blood triglycerides, and tissue damage from inflammation.[6]

Omega-3s Are Good for Your Gums

A study of nine thousand adults, ages 20 years and older, found that the rate of gum disease, or gingivitis, was 20 percent lower in people who reported consuming the most omega-3s.[7] Studies in animals show that DHA can reduce periodontitis.[8]

THE OMEGA-3 EFFECT: INFLAMMATORY BALANCE

Omegas in Balance	*Omegas Not in Balance*
• Blood vessels wide open (vasodilation)	• Blood vessels too narrow (vasoconstriction)
• Blood pressure stabilized	• Blood pressure too high
• Blood clotting just right	• Blood clotting too fast
• Bronchial airways wide open	• Airways constricted (asthma)
• Less pain in tissues	• Increased sensitivity to pain
• Increased protective mucus and decreased acid secretion in stomach	• Increased stomach acid production
• Enhanced healing	• Delayed healing

OMEGA-3S HELP BUILD HEALTHIER SKIN

Since most skin conditions are just another *-itis*, doctors can often guess whether the amount of omega-3s in a person's diet is sufficient by the feel of the person's skin.

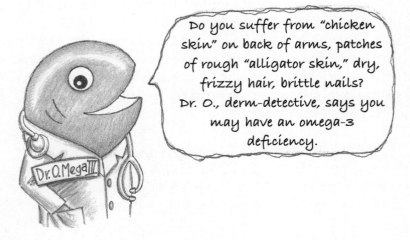

Do you suffer from "chicken skin" on back of arms, patches of rough "alligator skin," dry, frizzy hair, brittle nails? Dr. O., derm-detective, says you may have an omega-3 deficiency.

Taking omega-3 fish oil supplements and eating more seafood help you have healthier skin. Most skin conditions are due to inflammation. Omega-3s are natural anti-inflammatory oils. For over ten years, in my medical practice I've been prescribing fish oil for my patients with dry, scaly skin, eczema, psoriasis, and other forms of dermatitis. In the last few years, dermatologists have started doing the same, and science agrees.[9]

During routine checkups the look and feel of the skin often gives me a clue to how much omega-3 oil the patient eats. I look and feel for dry, rough skin as a possible sign of omega-3 deficiency. Since hair and nails come from the same embryological root cells as the skin, I also examine those tissues. When I see patients with eczema or dry, scaly skin, I ask them if they eat a lot of seafood or take fish oil supplements. They look surprised, probably wondering what fish has to do with their skin problems.

When treating dermatitis, I focus not only on the lotions and potions you put *onto* your skin but also the nutrients you put *into* your skin. That's where omega-3s shine. All that exposure to sun and wind, allergies, and the normal wear and tear of aging cause skin to lose its elasticity, wrinkle, become thinner and more sensitive to rashes.

Even babies get dermatitis (usually eczema), often caused by topical or food allergies or a genetic quirk. Skin at all ages loves omega-3s because omega-3 EPA/DHA is a smooth, soft, flexible nutrient that treats dermatitis from the inside. Studies reveal that when pregnant mothers eat more omega-3s and/or their infants eat more omega-3s, these babies experience less eczema.

A patient's letter to Dr. Bill:

In 1998 my baby was born with a rare genetic condition called congenital icthyosis (Greek for "fish skin"). Her skin was scaly. It bothered me more than her. At our two-week visit you surprised me by recommending I eat salmon two or three times a week and take fish oil supplements. You explained that the special fats would get into my breast milk and then into my baby's skin to help it heal. Within a month her skin was much smoother and softer, and her dermatologist at UCLA was amazed. Thank you, Dr. Sears!

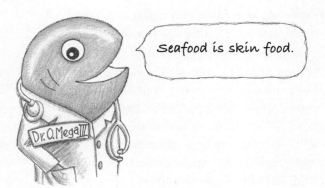

Seafood is skin food.

INFLAMMATION QUESTIONS YOU MAY HAVE

Happy Meals

I've heard of an anti-inflammatory diet. What is it?

Here's a simple anti-inflammatory diet I prescribe in our medical practice. I call it the five S's diet: seafood, salads, smoothies, spices, and supplements. I call these "happy meals" because not only are you happier when you're not hurting but neurological research is starting to reveal that the root cause of the chemical imbalances causing depression and other mood disorders may be inflammation or wear and tear on the nervous system. At least three times a week, eat happy meals — a fruit and yogurt smoothie in the morning and a multivegetable spicy salad topped with a salmon fillet for dinner. These anti-inflammatory powerhouses are just what the *-itis* doctor ordered. (For information about the "sipping solution" smoothie, see www.AskDrSears .com.)

Over-the-Counter Anti-Inflammatory Medications

What happens when I take anti-inflammatories such as aspirin and ibuprofen to relieve my joint pains?

Nonsteroidal anti-inflammatory drugs (NSAIDs) relieve the pain and swelling of inflammation. They are known as COX inhibitors, which means they partly suppress the production of the COX proinflammatory eicosanoids (see page 115). The problem with these COX inhibitors is that while they block pain, swelling, and blood clotting and can reduce the incidence of stroke and heart attacks, they can "overreact" by suppressing COX too much and actually cause bleeding, gastrointestinal upsets, and even heart attacks. This was the reason Vioxx was taken off the market in 2004. When you mess with Mother Nature, your body pays a price. To paraphrase advice from the omega researcher Dr. Bill Lands, instead of taking more drugs to kill excess COX chemicals, eat less omega-6 and more omega-3 to make a lower level of COX chemicals in your body.

Taking Omega-3s with NSAIDS

Should I take omega-3s with the NSAIDs my doctor recommended?

Absolutely! Because commercial anti-inflammatories inhibit both the good and the bad effects of inflammation, balance your inflammation by partnering these medications with fish oil. (See Chapter 11 for anti-inflammatory dosages.)

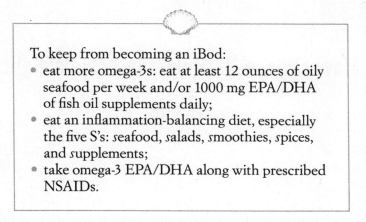

To keep from becoming an iBod:
- eat more omega-3s: eat at least 12 ounces of oily seafood per week and/or 1000 mg EPA/DHA of fish oil supplements daily;
- eat an inflammation-balancing diet, especially the five S's: *s*eafood, *s*alads, *s*moothies, *s*pices, and *s*upplements;
- take omega-3 EPA/DHA along with prescribed NSAIDs.

8

. . .

How Omega-3s Help You Lose Weight

What? Eat fat to lose fat? Yes. No other nutrient has been the subject of as much unscientific advice as fats. First came the low-fat diet craze. Dieters got fatter. Then came the hydrogenated fake fat fiasco, approved by the Food and Drug Administration and even endorsed by heart specialists ("eat margarine, not butter"). People got fatter—and sicker—before this factory-made fat was exposed for the sticky, sickie fat it is. Finally came the omega-3 oils, the most scientifically studied, healthiest oil on the planet. Yet, as of this writing, the U.S. Department of Agriculture (USDA) still has not issued an official Recommended Daily Intake (RDI) for omega-3s.

WHAT FATS MAKE YOU FAT?

After one of my "oil change" lectures in China, the discussion turned to the topic of obesity in the United States. Besides "portion distortion" (e.g., restaurant portions are large), a main contributor to the fattening of Americans is the shift in our diets to more fake factory food and less real food. Scientists who study the obesity epidemic have noticed that over the past thirty years weight and waist lines have increased together with the increase in factory-processed oils in the U.S. diet.[1] The increase in other packaged factory foods has clearly contributed to the rise in the obesity rate. Researchers who study obesity throughout the world have noted that people in cultures where diets are high in omega-3 EPA/DHA, such as in parts of Asia, tend not only to be healthier but leaner. Yet when they immigrate to the United States and start to eat fewer omega-3 oils and more factory-processed omega-6 oils, they get fatter.

Omega-3s are a lean food because they increase fat burning, decrease excess fat storage, improve satiety (curb overeating), and decrease the complications of obesity, such as inflammation and the metabolic syndrome.[2]

EAT MORE FISH, GET LESS FAT AND LESS SICK

Weight control doctors have concluded that eating more omega-3s helps with weight loss:

- When coastal dwellers, whose diet is naturally higher in seafood, move inland and live off the land instead of the sea, they tend to lose their leanness.
- People with low blood levels of omega-3 EPA/DHA tend to have a greater risk of the metabolic syndrome: high body mass index, large waist size, high blood pressure, high blood sugar, and high blood cholesterol and triglycerides.[3]
- Some weight loss programs that combine fish oil with exercise reduce more body fat.[4]
- Studies analyzing children's diets revealed that those with the highest body mass index had the highest omega-6 and the lowest omega-3 blood levels.[5]

While omega-3 supplements by themselves don't qualify as a weight loss supplement, there is plenty of science to support that they do reduce the complications of obesity, mainly inflammation. Fat cells called adipocytes, especially in excess belly fat, release into the bloodstream potent proinflammatory chemicals called adipokines, which promote *-itis* illnesses. Omega-3s help blunt the tissue damage from an excess of inflammation-causing chemicals.

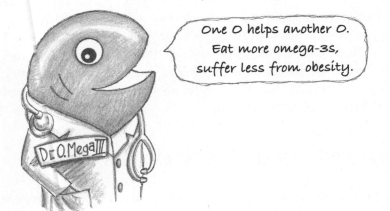

One O helps another O. Eat more omega-3s, suffer less from obesity.

SEAFOOD IS MORE FILLING, LESS FATTENING

Seafood is a high-satiety food. One of the reasons that omega-3s are appropriately called a lean fat is that they make you feel full with less food. Because seafood is so nutrient-dense (packed with lots of nutrition per calorie), you are satisfied with fewer calories.[6] Try this feel-better-after-eating experiment. First, eat a 6-ounce salmon fillet. Notice how your gut feels shortly after the meal and two or three hours later. If your gut could talk, it would say, "I feel good, as a gut should, and I'm so satisfied, not uncomfortably full nor hungry." On another day eat the same number of calories in a high-carbohydrate meal, say, pasta. Notice how your gut feels. You will probably feel hungrier sooner, even though you ate the same number of calories as in your seafood meal.

Why these different gut feelings? Unlike seafood, carbohydrates have a low satiety factor. When you're less satisfied, or even hungry, you tend to crave and eat more carbs and get fatter.

The next day eat a 6-ounce sirloin steak, and listen to your gut saying, "I don't feel good, as a gut should." You may feel too full too fast, constipated, and lethargic as the blood reluctantly diverts from brain to gut to help process the overload. You just experienced a case of postprandial lipemia (PPL), or high blood levels of sticky fats after a meal. (See more about PPL, page 54.)

In a 2008 study, scientists discovered that people who ate a diet containing more than 1300 mg of omega-3s per day (about 4 ounces of oily fish) felt more comfortably full sooner, compared with people who ate low omega-3 meals (less than 260 mg per day).[7] The researchers concluded that a diet with a high level of omega-3 fats should be standard in a successful weight loss program. Called postprandial satiety, or after-meal fullness, this may explain how a meal rich in omega-3s helps to curb overeating.

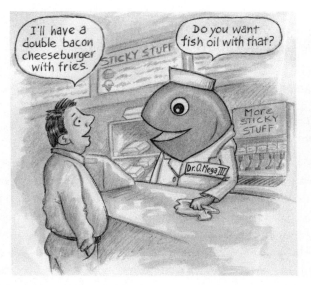

SHOCKING STATISTICS

Did you know that childhood obesity is now one of the most serious diseases in many countries throughout the world? In 2005 the Centers for Disease Control and Prevention issued a statement that shook many parents into a kitchen makeover: "Unless American families change the way they eat and live, one in three children will grow up to be diabetic." Because the casual advice, "Oh, he's just overweight; he'll grow out of it," wasn't working, pediatricians have had to strengthen their language. I no longer use the word *overweight*. Instead, I say to parents, "Your child is *prediabetic*." That gets their attention, and families will start to change their habits, especially by eating more omega-3s.

This could explain why people in cultures that eat a seafood-rich diet, such as the Japanese, tend to be leaner and healthier than those who eat less seafood and more carbohydrates.

WEIGHT LOSS QUESTIONS YOU MAY HAVE

Supplements Instead of Seafood?

I don't like fish. Would just taking fish oil supplements help me lose weight?

Probably not. While omega-3 supplements may reduce some of the complications of obesity, such as inflammation, for optimal weight control I advise eating more seafood *plus* taking a fish oil supplement. In fact, a 2011 study showed that taking a high-dose fish oil supplement alone did not lead to weight loss.[8] Waist watchers, I don't want you to believe that all you have to do to lose excess body fat is to pop a daily fish oil pill. Giving yourself the right oil change is just one of many changes necessary to get lean and stay lean. (For information about the L.E.A.N. program for general health and weight control, see www.DrSearsLean.com.)

Toxic Waist

I'm eating more seafood and less junk food.
I've gone down two belt notches, but my weight
hasn't changed much. Help!

Reducing your *waist* is more healthful medically than reducing your *weight*. Excess abdominal flab is literally a "different animal" than the excess fat in your cheeks, thighs, and buttocks. The fat cells in belly flab become a chemical factory spewing into your bloodstream anti-medicines, harmful chemicals that increase your chances of cardiovascular disease, diabetes, cancer, and many *-itis* illnesses. This is why doctors are putting more emphasis on *waist* reduction rather than just *weight* reduction.

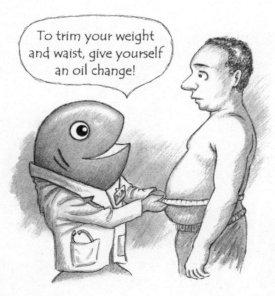

I was explaining "waist management" to one of my portly patients, who quipped, "The next time we meet, you will see less of me."

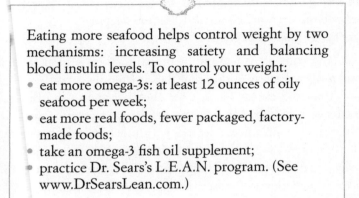

Eating more seafood helps control weight by two mechanisms: increasing satiety and balancing blood insulin levels. To control your weight:
- eat more omega-3s: at least 12 ounces of oily seafood per week;
- eat more real foods, fewer packaged, factory-made foods;
- take an omega-3 fish oil supplement;
- practice Dr. Sears's L.E.A.N. program. (See www.DrSearsLean.com.)

9

. . .

How Omega-3s Help Keep You Young

"Welcome, prime-timers!" I surprised and pleased an audience during an omega-3 talk one evening. They liked this title better than "seniors." My interest in eating more omega-3s to stay younger began with my research discovering that people in cultures that eat the most omega-3s live the longest and healthiest and remain the smartest.

WHAT'S IN YOUR BODY AND BRAIN BANK?

One of the best nutritional investments you can make into your IRAH (Individual Retirement Account for Health) is to start young to deposit high doses of omega-3s into your tissues. The higher the tissue levels of omega-3s, the healthier nearly every organ will continue to be.

A recent birthday card I received from my son read, "Getting older isn't so bad when you consider the alternative." This is true, which is why I don't like the term *anti-aging*. We can't actually stop aging, but we *can* slow aging and often even reverse some disease effects of aging.

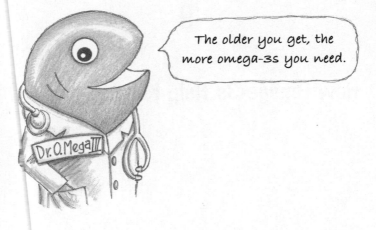

The older you get, the more omega-3s you need.

Dr. O. Mega III

WHY WE AGE: SCIENCE MADE SIMPLE

Here's a simple definition of aging; I call it inflam-aging: Sticky stuff (inflammation) accumulates in your tissues. Aging results from wear and tear on tissues, caused mostly by accumulation of sticky stuff. Again, the tissue is the issue. What's the top anti-inflammatory nutrient? Omega-3 EPA/DHA. With aging, cell membranes gradually lose some of their fluidity and become stiffer. Omega-3s help improve cell membrane fluidity. And according to neuroscientists, levels of omega-3s in brain tissue may decline with age,[1] another reason we need to eat more omega-3s as we age. So I believe, and science supports, that omega-3s are the top foods for healthy aging. Here's why science and common sense say we prime-timers need to eat more sea-food. Notice how omega-3 EPA/DHA helps nearly every aging process that's going on in your body.

Why Seniors Need More Seafood

What Happens as You Age	How Omega-3 EPA/DHA Can Help
The -*itis* illnesses become more common.	Potent anti-inflammatory effect reduces -*itis* illnesses (see Chapter 7).
Blood vessel walls become stiff, and sticky stuff accumulates on their lining, narrowing arteries, raising blood pressure, and weakening the heart muscle.	Vessels dilate, vessel walls and lining stay smooth and soft, blood pressure stays normal, and heart muscle stays strong.[2]
Blood tends to overclot, causing thrombosis and stroke.	Natural anticoagulant effect prevents blood from clotting too fast and lessens chance of stroke.[3]
Brain tissue shrinks, and nerve transmission slows. Sticky stuff accumulates from inflammation, and Alzheimer's disease can develop.	Myelin and brain cell membranes stay strong, inflammation lessens, thinking stays sharp.[4]
Brain tissue levels of omega-3 DHA naturally decline.	Slows cognitive decline.[5]
Dementia and depression increase.	Stabilizes moods.[6]
Retinal vessels narrow. Macular degeneration develops.	Retinal tissue vessels stay open, and less sticky stuff accumulates. May protect against macular degeneration.[7]
Gums get inflamed and weaken.	Helps prevent gingivitis.[8]
Skin gets inflamed, rough, and wrinkly.	Helps prevent dryness, wrinkles, and dermatitis (see Chapter 7).

(continued)

What Happens as You Age	How Omega-3 EPA/DHA Can Help
Immunity weakens.	Strengthens immunity (see Chapter 7).
Joints stiffen and arthritis results.	Joints stay mobile (see Chapter 7).
Hearing loss occurs.	Delays age-related hearing loss.[9]
Bones get frail.	Helps increase bone mineral density.[10]

FOR LONGEVITY, GO FISH!

A 2008 study showed that in 254 patients with an average age of 82 those who ate the most fish and had the highest levels of omega-3 EPA lived the longest.[11] When it comes to healthy aging, in addition to helping your heart, omega-3s are the fats that help keep your brain smart. In fact, the three areas of your body these fats help the most are your brain, your heart, and your joints. Eating more omega-3 EPA/DHA has been shown to help with nearly all the ailments of aging, especially cardiovascular disease, rheumatoid arthritis, Crohn's disease, ulcerative colitis, dermatitis, lupus, and Alzheimer's disease. (For information on omega-3s and Alzheimer's disease, see page 78.)

Top Off Your Telomeres. A new way of measuring biological aging is telomere length. Telomeres "bind up" the ends of chromosomes, like the tip of a shoelace. As we age, these telomeres are gradually snipped shorter. Researchers who study aging use telomere length at the cellular level as a marker of general health and how fast a person is aging. People with slower telomere shortening tend to age more slowly.[12] When the chromosomes of 608 seniors were studied over a five-year period, those who enjoyed the highest blood levels of omega-3 EPA/DHA tended to have longer telomeres.[13] Researchers concluded that this genetic perk may be one of the reasons that

SCIENCE SAYS: SLOW AGING, BE HAPPY

Many seniors suffer from depression. What's more, the side effects of antidepressant drugs tend to be more severe the older we get. Unlike prescription mood-mellowing medicines that offer little help but lots of harm, omega-3 EPA/DHA (1000–2500 mg of fish oil daily) tends to provide some relief from depression in seniors.

people who eat more omega-3s enjoy healthier aging. A 2008 study coauthored by my friend Dr. Dean Ornish showed that patients who improved their diet and lifestyle increased their telomere-lengthening enzymes nearly 30 percent within three months.[14]

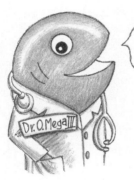

> My wish for healthy aging: Everything works and nothing hurts.

HEALTHY AGING QUESTIONS YOU MAY HAVE

Nursing Home Nutrition

My 85-year-old mother is in a nursing home.
How can I help her make healthy changes?

Let me tell you about my nursing home experience with my own mother. When I saw the food my mother was being served, I was shocked. The very age group who needed the best food was fed the worst food. So, like a good doctor and good son, I made an "instead of" list. Instead of "old foods," those that worsened my mother's health, I insisted she get "young foods" to nourish her health.

OLD FOODS VS. YOUNG FOODS

Instead of	Eat
• Fatty meat	• Seafood
• White bread	• 100% whole grains
• Processed and hydrogenated oils	• Olive oil, flax oil
• Cereals, artificially colored or sweetened	• Eggs
• Yogurt with artificial fillers and sweeteners	• Greek yogurt sweetened with blueberries
• Iceberg lettuce	• Spinach
• Fatty gravy and sauces	• Olive oil and balsamic vinegar, spices like turmeric, cinnamon
• Three big meals a day	• Six minimeals a day
• Forks for large mouthfuls	• An option: chopsticks for smaller bites and slower eating, and to build extra brain-cell connections

When I presented my healthy aging eating changes to the nursing home, I received a not-so-surprising excuse: "Dr. Sears, medically we agree with your changes, but we can't afford the extra costs. Medicare only pays us so much." Oh, that cost-cutting excuse again, I thought. Spend less on food but spend much more on hospital and drug costs. Hippocrates exposed this fallacy over two thousand years ago, and we still don't get it.

Here are some tips to help keep your parents young at heart, mind, and body. As always, consult a physician before making any change in dietary or health plans:

- Give them this book to read, especially this chapter.
- Bring them a home-cooked seafood dinner, or take them to a seafood restaurant twice a week.
- Bring them omega-3 supplements equivalent to 500 mg daily of EPA/DHA. Eating omega-3s both in seafood and supplement form would ensure they get sufficient amounts.
- Try to get the menu makers at the nursing home to serve more safe seafood and other whole foods and less sticky stuff, and tell them it will make their patient care easier.
- Use liquid fish oils if capsules are too big to swallow.

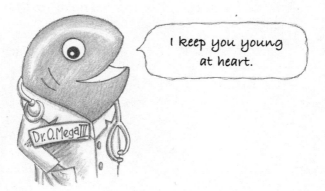

Healthy Aging Plan

Besides eating more omega-3s, what else can I do to lessen my chances of getting sick as I get older?

This is a question I asked myself in my fifties. So Martha and I put together a healthy aging plan in my book *Prime-Time Health*

(Little, Brown, 2010). This plan is also on DVD: *9 Simple Steps to Prime-Time Health,* available at www.AskDrSears.com. The main theme of our organ-by-organ health plan is to show you how to tap into your own personal pharmacy and help your body make its own internal medicines.

For healthy aging:
- eat at least 12 ounces of oily seafood weekly, or eat at least 1000 mgs of omega-3 EPA/DHA fish oil supplements daily;
- eat more real foods, fewer processed foods;
- eat more of the five S's: seafood, salads, smoothies, spices, supplements;
- graze: eat by the rule of 2s: twice as often, half as much, chew twice as long.

10

. . .

How Omega-3s Help You Heal

One day while making hospital rounds I wondered, If hospitals are where healing occurs, and omega-3s are natural healers, why is the standard hospital diet deficient in omega-3s? It's a rerun of the standard American diet (SAD), which is what puts many patients in the hospital in the first place. After all, if hospitals believe that food is medicine, the food they serve should have medicinal qualities. But my first impression of the food destined for delivery to unsuspecting sick patients was, low-budget airline food: fatty sauces and meats, artificially sweetened and colored cereals, yogurt, and gelatin desserts.

Where's the fish? I wondered. Seafood should be hospital food.

As a doctor I was ashamed of this omega deficiency in the very kitchen that should be serving at least an omega-3-sufficient diet or, even better, a diet high in healing omega-3 fats.[1]

While writing this book, I had the experience of helping two of my favorite patients heal with the help of omega-3s.

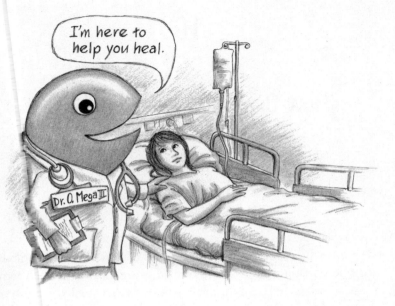

Hospital Food Should Be Healing Food

Patients' Problem	Omega-3 Helpful Effect
Inflammation, -itis illness	Anti-inflammatory effect
Thrombosis: heart attack, stroke	Regulates blood clotting
Infection	Boosts immunity
Wound	Heals tissues
Allergic illness	Anti-allergic benefit
Hormonal imbalance	Hormonal harmony
Depression, mood disorder	Antidepressant effect
Nerve damage	Regenerates nerve tissue
Fracture	Heals bone
Heart surgery	Helps prevent arrhythmia
Longer hospital stay	Shortens hospital stay

TRAUMATIZED TISSUES HEALED FASTER

My first story is about Shane, whom I have cared for since birth. Shane, 11 years old, had suffered a bad injury to his leg from a boating accident, and he needed a lot of reconstructive surgery. Remembering my omega-3 mantra—The tissue is the issue— that's what I prescribed. I loaded Shane up with salmon and fish oil for weeks after his injury, and he healed faster than any of his surgeons had predicted.

BRAIN SURGERY HEALED FASTER

My second story is about our 15-year-old grandson, Alex. We learned that Alex was diagnosed with a brain tumor. Fortunately, it was not malignant. Unfortunately, it was located in the most vulnerable part of the brain, the brain stem. Adjacent to this growing tumor was a major artery to the brain stem as well as some major nerves to the rest of the body. This type of tumor is called "malignant by position," meaning that while it doesn't metastasize to other parts of the body, it can eventually damage adjacent vital brain tissue as it grows. Within a couple of months he would need, according to the surgeon, "major brain surgery, possibly lasting as long as fifteen hours."

A few days after the diagnosis, I sat with Alex and his parents and outlined what I called his personal pre-op and post-op program. We all wanted Alex's body and brain at their best during the operation and for optimal healing afterward. Since Alex wanted to know more about how foods, especially omega-3s, help brain tissue heal, I advised him to eat the following:

- *A right-fat diet.* Brain tissue is 60 percent fat. Therefore, a patient recovering from major brain surgery (healing, swelling, inflammation, infection) needs to eat good fats, such as seafood, ground flaxseeds, avocado, and olive oil.

- *A healing diet.* A post-op surgical patient needs to control inflammation and infection and enhance wound healing. Therefore, the healing tissues need foods that promote, rather than interfere with, healing, especially the five S's: seafood, (fruit) smoothies, salads, spices, and supplements. I recommended that besides eating more of these, Alex take extra antioxidants in a nutritional supplement called Juice Plus, which is a concentrated fruit-and-vegetable extract in a capsule.

- *A nerve-regrowth diet.* To help the nervous tissue affected by the surgery regenerate, the patient needs foods that grow new nerves, make myelin, promote synaptic connections and proper synaptic firing, decrease inflammation, and suppress infection. Brain cells have the most mitochondria (tiny areas in the cell that act like storage batteries that produce energy). Because brain cells are one of the highest energy-producing tissues, they generate the most free radicals (also called oxidants or wear and tear chemicals) from biochemical exhaust. Therefore, brain cells need more antioxidants to help them grow and heal. That's one of the ways omega-3s help brain tissue heal.

- *A gut-soothing diet.* Because the gut flora (natural bacteria) have been compromised by the necessary use of broad-spectrum antibiotics to prevent post-op infections, the gut needs replenishing by probiotics (yogurt bacteria) and pre-biotics (foods that feed the natural bacteria).

Superintelligent and supermotivated, Alex got the connection between how he eats and how he heals.

My first prescription was a box of salmon fillets from the Sears family fish freezer. (When our monthly "catch" arrives by FedEx from my favorite seafood source, Vitalchoice.com, Martha announces, "Bill, your medicine has arrived.") My instructions to Alex: "Eat six ounces of salmon four times a week."

This dose would give Alex at least 1000 mg of omega-3 DHA/EPA per day, which is a sufficient dose for any school-age child, teen, or adult, but he might need a higher dose to help him heal. Since the main issue was to heal brain tissue, I told Alex "go fish" would be the two important dietary words before and after his operation.

Omega-3s are to brain tissue what calcium and vitamin D are to the bones. As you would be advised to take more calcium and vitamin D during healing from a fracture, you should take more omega-3s to help brain tissue heal. Salmon provides the triple whammy of being high in omega-3s, vitamin D, and calcium. Canned salmon with the soft cooked bones is the highest in calcium. I consider wild Alaskan sockeye salmon to be one of the top healing foods because its pink color indicates a naturally occurring powerful antioxidant and immune booster called astaxanthin. (For more about astaxanthin, see page 180.)

ADAPTOGENS

Biochemically, the healing molecules in fish oil are called adaptogens, meaning they get into the tissues to heal them and bring them back to normal but don't cause disease. An example of this adaptogen effect is that fish oil can lower high blood pressure in people who have high blood pressure but does not affect the blood pressure of people with normal blood pressure.

BRAIN TRAUMA HEALED FASTER

To further drive home the healing power of omega-3s, I'd like to tell you about the coal miner Randal McCloy, who was rescued after being trapped two miles underground in a collapsed coal mine for forty-one hours. His twelve fellow miners had already perished from carbon monoxide poisoning. Heart barely beating and nearly brain-dead, McCloy was rushed to West Virginia University Hospital, where the neurosurgeon Julian Bailes was called upon to bring McCloy's carbon monoxide (CO)–poisoned brain back to health.

Prolonged oxygen deprivation and CO exposure damage the fatty layer of brain cell nerve tissue (myelin), the insulating covering that enables nerve messages to travel so fast. It follows that injured myelin is damaged fat. What does injured fat need? Oxygen and healthy fat. Dr. Bailes placed his patient in a hyperbaric oxygen room and prescribed 15 000 mg (15 grams) of omega-3 EPA/DHA fish oil per day. That's equivalent to around 4 pounds of salmon in one sitting, about five times the usually recommended therapeutic dose of omega-3s for neurological diseases.

After a few weeks, McCloy awakened from his coma. Within a few more weeks he further astonished his medical team by walking, talking, and recovering his memory.

When *Men's Health* interviewed Dr. Bailes, the neurosurgeon explained, "The omega-3s helped rebuild the damaged gray and white matter of his brain."[2] McCloy continued to follow his doctor's orders by taking daily fish oil supplements, and his nerve tissue function continued to improve.

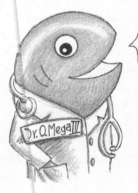

The fishier the meal, the better you heal.

Fish oil therapy may soon be coming to a hospital near you. An omega-3 Top Doc, Robert Martingale, MD, PhD (nutrition), chief of surgery and director of nutritional services at Oregon Health and Science University, revealed that omega-3 therapy is as potent as some drugs. Dr. Martingale stated that he routinely prescribes fish oil supplementation for five days prior to elective surgery. He added that the Society for Critical Care Medicine has given fish oil therapy its highest scientific rating — grade A — for use in critical care management. And he calmed some critics by assuring that in his studies high doses of fish oil did not cause dangerous post-op bleeding. At a conference on Nutritional Armor for the Warfighter, he spoke of new research on injecting fish oil intravenously at the time of injury to speed recovery.[3]

OMEGA-3S: NUTRITIONAL ARMOR FOR THE MILITARY

In 2009 military health care providers and omega-3 researchers came together at a conference on Nutritional Armor for the Warfighter: Can Omega-3 Fatty Acids Enhance Stress Resilience, Wellness, and Military Performance? After summarizing the science, experts including former Surgeon General Richard Carmona, MD, and Captain Joseph Hibbeln, MD, came to the conclusion that science supports that sufficient omega-3s are necessary to optimize the wellness and performance of our warriors.[4] They further concluded that omega-3s should be considered one of many medicines in the prevention and treatment of military-related illnesses. It was refreshing to hear these respected scientists and medical doctors refer to omega-3s as medicines. Dr. Carmona revealed his frustration that the overwhelming science supporting the healing powers of omega-3s has not been appreciated enough. "How much data do you need before you act?" he said.

In discussing the science demonstrating that omega-3s help warriors handle stress, Dr. Hibbeln revealed that four out of every ten military hospital beds are occupied by soldiers suffering from a combat-stress-related psychiatric illness, and omega-3s can help: "When the brain is deficient in omega-3s, it's like the foot is heavy on the emotional gas petal and not on the brake when it needs to be," he said.

MEDICAL QUESTIONS YOU MAY HAVE

Consult Your Surgeon First

I'm having elective surgery in a few weeks,
and I take omega-3 supplements. Should
I consult my surgeon?

An understandable concern that some surgeons may have is the possible anticoagulating effect of omega-3s, which may cause the surgical site to bleed during or after the operation. This has been thoroughly addressed and researched, and at a dose of 1000 mg of omega-3 EPA/DHA per day there should be no increased bleeding tendency. This is equivalent to the average omega-3 intake of eating 6 ounces of salmon four times per week. In fact, the Food and Drug Administration has issued a recommendation not to exceed 3000 mg per day if increased bleeding is a concern. I believe, and research supports, that depending on a patient's age, serving a pre-op and post-op patient 6 ounces of wild salmon three to four times per week is in the safe and therapeutic range. Since the concern about increased bleeding is a possible trade-off for increased healing, naturally it would need to be discussed with your doctor.

Snake Oil?

*My friend's doctor called my fish oil supplements
"snake oil." What should I say?*

I recently encountered this criticism from a cardiologist caring
for one of my patients in the hospital. Not only is there more scientific support for the healing properties of fish oil than for many
of the prescription medicines in the hospital pharmacy, the original snake oil has actually been shown to have high healing properties. At one time this reptile oil was vilified as pseudoscience or
quackery. New research, however, has raised snake oil to some
respectability by showing it contains tissue-healing enzymes,
such as phospholipase A2. The rattler muscle in rattlesnakes, a
high-contraction-frequency muscle, is high in omega-3 DHA.[5]

Following is the handout I give my patients who are preparing
to undergo a major medical or surgical procedure. Feeding
patients lots of healing foods before a major surgical procedure is
called *preloading* with nutrients.

FISH OIL SAVES BABIES' LIVERS AND LIVES

At the 2012 GOED conference, doctors presented therapeutic
uses for fish oil not only to help patients heal from TBI (Traumatic
Brain Injury) but also in TPN (Total Parenteral Nutrition). Pediatric surgeons at Boston Children's Hospital showed how infants
who were treated with sufficient doses of fish oil healed faster
from liver failure. Because fish oil was not yet FDA approved for
this treatment, these doctors were granted a "compassionate use"
exemption, which they believed saved many lives.

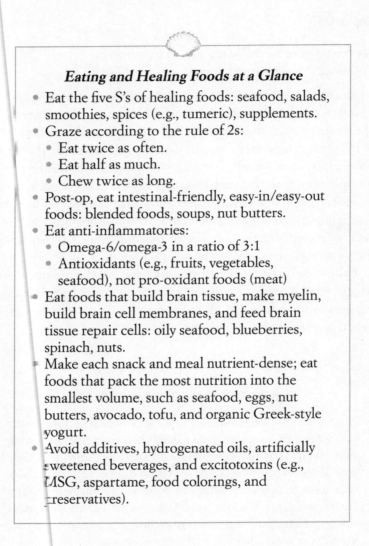

Eating and Healing Foods at a Glance

- Eat the five S's of healing foods: seafood, salads, smoothies, spices (e.g., tumeric), supplements.
- Graze according to the rule of 2s:
  - Eat twice as often.
  - Eat half as much.
  - Chew twice as long.
- Post-op, eat intestinal-friendly, easy-in/easy-out foods: blended foods, soups, nut butters.
- Eat anti-inflammatories:
  - Omega-6/omega-3 in a ratio of 3:1
  - Antioxidants (e.g., fruits, vegetables, seafood), not pro-oxidant foods (meat)
- Eat foods that build brain tissue, make myelin, build brain cell membranes, and feed brain tissue repair cells: oily seafood, blueberries, spinach, nuts.
- Make each snack and meal nutrient-dense; eat foods that pack the most nutrition into the smallest volume, such as seafood, eggs, nut butters, avocado, tofu, and organic Greek-style yogurt.
- Avoid additives, hydrogenated oils, artificially sweetened beverages, and excitotoxins (e.g., MSG, aspartame, food colorings, and preservatives).

SELECTING FISH OIL SUPPLEMENTS AND ENJOYING SAFE SEAFOOD

An omega-3 deficiency is the top nutritional deficiency in the United States. Most Americans, at all ages, eat only 20 percent of the daily omega-3s they need. Data from the U.S. Department of Agriculture reveal that Americans eat only an average of 3½ ounces of seafood weekly, far short of the recommended 12 ounces per week. To point out how omega-3 EPA/DHA is deficient in the typical Western diet: children eating the standard American diet (SAD) average only 19 mg omega-3 DHA per day. Pregnant mothers average only 120 mg omega-3 per day. Adult Americans average 150 mg of omega-3s per day, Europeans average 300 mg per day, and Japanese average nearly 1000 mg per day. It's no surprise we are a sick society, spending more on medical care per person than any country in the world. According to recent data from the Chinese Nutrition Society, the Chinese average only 37 mg of omega-3s per day.[1] This is one reason I've been invited to lecture in China on increasing dietary intake of omega-3s.

The following chapters explain how to select fish oil supplements that are right for you, and how to shop for safe seafood, those fish that have the most omega-3s and lowest amount of mercury. I also give some cooking tips to make your family's meals more delicious and nutritious. After reading these chapters you will truly want to go fish!

11

. . .

Getting the Most Omega-3 Effect out of Omega-3 Supplements

Now that you know why omega-3s are a top nutrient for head-to-toe health, I summarize the best available science to prescribe the right dosage for ailments you have or don't want to get, and I answer other omega-3 questions you may have.

Based on information from trusted scientific sources, for most adults I recommend eating

---

1000 milligrams (mg) per day of omega-3 EPA/DHA

Note that in this chapter "milligrams per day" means milligrams per day of *omega-3 EPA and DHA,* not milligrams of fish oil, since there are other omegas in fish oil. (See how to read a fish oil supplement label, page 158.)

You will notice that my dosage recommendations may be higher than others you read. Here are the questions I asked to arrive at the recommended numbers.

HOW MUCH OMEGA-3 SHOULD HEALTHY PEOPLE EAT?

How much omega-3 do the healthiest world cultures eat? The Japanese, who enjoy the longest health span and life span in the world, eat an average of 700–1000 mg omega-3 EPA/DHA per day.

What dosages do the top scientists recommend? My recommendations generally follow those of the International Society for the Study of Fatty Acids and Lipids, the National Institutes of Health, the American Heart Association, and the Institute of Medicine.

CONSULT YOUR DOCTOR FIRST

Before taking more than 1000 milligrams (mg) per day of omega-3 DHA/EPA fish oil supplements, check with your health care provider. Even though science says higher dosages are safe, you may have a special metabolic quirk that requires special attention to dosing.

Minimum Dose for Adults

The minimum dose of omega-3 EPA/DHA for adults is as follows [1]

- Fish oil supplements: 500 mg per day per 2000 calories consumed, or
- Oily seafood: 12 ounces per week (equals 500–600 mg per day depending on the species)

My personal recommendation is that rather than taking the minimum of 500 mg, most healthy adults should try to get

1000 mg (1 gram) per day of omega-3 EPA/DHA. You can get this amount by eating 12 ounces per week of safe seafood and/or 500–1000 mg per day fish oil supplements, depending on how much seafood you eat.

DO YOUR OWN DOSAGE MATH

Omega-3 experts calculate that the healthy models for daily omega-3 consumption are the Japanese and Greenlanders, who eat nearly 0.4 percent of their daily calories in the form of omega-3 fats, mostly from marine sources.[2] Practically, this translates to about 1000 mg omega-3 fats per 2000 calories per day.

So, an active person burning 3000 calories per day would need about 1500 mg of omega-3 fats daily. A person burning 1500 calories would need about 750 mg of omega-3 fats daily.

Minimum Dose for Adults with Heart Disease

The minimum dose of omega-3 EPA/DHA for adults with heart disease is 1000 mg per day.

Minimum Dose for Infants and Children

The minimum dose of omega-3 EPA/DHA for infants and children is as follows:

- Infants: 300 mg per day
- Children, ages 2–3 years: 420 mg per day
- Children, ages 3 years and up: at least 500 mg per day

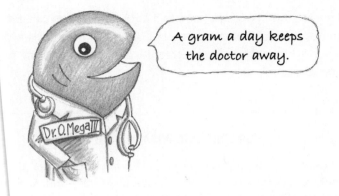

HOW MUCH OMEGA-3 FOR VARIOUS ILLNESSES?

The general recommendation of 500 mg EPA/DHA per day per 2000 calories consumed is the *minimum* preventive medicine dosage. Here are the dosage ranges for adults with various illnesses.

Dose for Neurological Disorders

Adults with neurological disorders like depression or bipolar disorders should take at least 2000 mg (2 grams) per day of EPA in a fish oil supplement. To this I add, eat 12 ounces of oily fish per week. Depending on the severity of your diagnosis, your doctor may adjust the dose. Neurological studies have used dosages ranging from 2000 mg to 6000 mg (2 to 6 grams) of omega-3 EPA/DHA per day, either EPA alone or EPA in combination with a lesser amount of DHA.

Dose for Cardiovascular Disease

The American Heart Association recommends that adults who have cardiovascular disease, or a high risk for it, eat *at least* 1000 mg omega-3 EPA/DHA daily.[3] How much omega-3 EPA/DHA to take depends upon the type and severity of the heart problem you have. My personal recommendation is to eat 6 ounces of wild salmon four times per week. Depending on the species of seafood, this would give you at least 1000–1200 mg of omega-3 EPA/DHA per day. (See Appendixes B and C for the omega-3 content of various seafoods.)

OPTIMAL NUTRITIONAL ALLOWANCE

Think ONA, not RDA. The older term, RDA (recommended daily allowance), means the minimum daily value of a nutrient to prevent disease. The newer term, ONA (optimal nutritional allowance), means the amount of a daily nutrient necessary for most people to give them the best health. The lower dosage of omega-3s that you still see in some government recommendations (e.g., 250 mg per day) represents the RDA. The dosages advised in this book are the optimal nutritional allowance.

Now, I realize many of you don't like to eat that much fish and prefer fish oil supplements. You could take 1000 mg of omega-3 EPA/DHA fish oil supplements per day plus two 6-ounce servings of oily fish per week, for a total of 2000 mg per day.

For people with very high triglyceride levels, the American Heart Association recommends up to 4000 mg omega-3 EPA/DHA per day, which may lower high triglyceride levels by 30–40 percent.[4]

Dose for -*itis* Illnesses

The dosage varies according to your -*itis* illness. Generally, it's 3000–4000 mg (3–4 grams) per day. For arthritis, science suggests the 3 + 3 guideline: 3000 mg (3 grams) per day for three months.[5] It often takes three months for people suffering from arthritis to experience the optimal omega-3 effect, after which the dose can be tapered down.

THE MEAL EFFECT

To improve the absorption of fish oil supplements, take them with a meal that contains healthy fats.

DOSAGE-SELECTING QUESTIONS YOU MAY HAVE

DHA and/or EPA?

As an omega-3 newbie, I take omega-3 supplements, but I'm confused. Some have only DHA, others DHA and EPA. Which is better?

For the past decade, scientists who study omega-3 fats have wondered which omega-3 is more important, DHA or EPA, and whether it is okay to take a supplement of one but not the other. Although DHA is present in brain tissue in much higher amounts than EPA, it's vital to eat both. EPA supports brain health by enhancing blood vessel health and blood flow to the brain. We know from studies that when you eat EPA, the brain rapidly gobbles it up, so the brain must need it to protect itself from inflammation. Again, when in doubt, take a tip from my favorite scientist, Mother Nature.

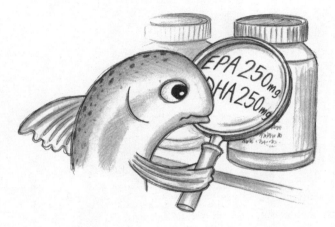

Fish Have Both Omega-3s. Omega-3 EPA/DHA is naturally found in certain fish, such as sockeye salmon, in a 1:1.4 ratio, with the proportion of DHA being slightly higher than that of EPA. Even algae, one of the most abundant seafoods that fish eat, contains both DHA and EPA. In fact, most fish contain an EPA/DHA ratio of about 1:1 or 1:2.

Mother's Milk Has Both Omega-3s. Both EPA and DHA occur naturally in mother's milk in a ratio that varies according to her diet. When mom eats fish or takes fish oils containing various omega-3 EPA and DHA ratios, her mammary glands sort out what's right for mother and baby. Breast milk always contains both DHA and EPA, with a slightly higher proportion of DHA.

So if both EPA and DHA are in the fish that swim in the sea and in the milk that mothers make, the perfect food for their babies, it seems prudent to conclude that we should eat both. The illustration shows what you should look for on a fish oil label.

Some nutritional supplements, especially those intended for infants and children, contain DHA only, and that's okay, for two reasons. First, in the early years it seems that DHA is the preferred omega-3 because children are in the stage of rapid brain growth.

At one time it was thought that only DHA was important because it is the omega-3 that predominates in nervous tissue, such as the brain, which contains very little EPA. But studies by Dr. Joseph Hibbeln at the National Institutes of Health showed that when the blood-brain barrier is injured and needs healing, it's EPA that comes to the rescue as part of healing the inflammation. Also, the brain is a very vascular organ. EPA is vital for vascular health.

While it's smart to eat both EPA and DHA, there is no need to worry whether you may be deficient in one or the other as long as you eat sufficient omega-3s. Mother Nature has a protective biochemical process called interconversion. DHA can be enzymatically converted to EPA and, to a lesser extent, vice versa, so that your tissues get whichever of these vital fats they most need. Yet, because scientists are still trying to pin down the exact percentage of interconversion of these two fatty acids, it's still best to eat both, since the rate of interconversion may vary from person to person.

CONSIDER THE CONCEPT OF SYNERGY

EPA and DHA are close friends. They work together. Synergy means that when one friend joins hands with another friend, their powers are multiplied, as if 1 + 1 = 3 or 4 or more. While EPA has its own unique benefits, it helps its friend DHA work better. Since EPA and DHA are buddies always found together, it makes sense to eat them together. EPA and DHA really show their synergy in the cell membrane. An important function of DHA is as a structural component of the human cell membrane, while EPA, by reducing the risk of inflammation, acts as a sort of cell maintenance engineer to protect cell function. DHA is the most abundant fatty acid in the brain and retina, but EPA still has a role in keeping excessive brain inflammation in check. Basically, EPA keeps the balance between tissue wear and tear and repair.

Omega-3 Blood Level

Is there a blood test I can get that measures how high my levels of omega-3s are?

Yes. In addition to the standard blood lipid analysis for cholesterol and triglycerides, an omega profile is now available. I believe it should be included as part of the standard blood tests when assessing your risk of cardiovascular disease. Because tissue levels of omega-3s are more relevant than blood levels, new tests measure your tissue levels. Since the easiest tissue to obtain is red blood cell membranes, ask your doctor to order a "red blood cell membrane omega-3 level." These blood tests measure both your red blood cell omega-3 percentage and the omega-6/omega-3 ratio as well as levels of other fatty acids in the red cell membranes. The percentage of omega-3s in red blood cell membranes accurately mirrors that of brain and heart tissue.

The higher the amount of omega-3s in your red blood cell membranes, the lower your risk of cardiovascular disease. A measurement of 8 percent or higher is the cardioprotective level to aim for. If you consume an average of 1000–1500 mg of omega-3 EPA/DHA per day (from seafood and/or supplements), you should be able to achieve this desirable level within a few months. My most recent level was 10.4 percent. The Japanese average is 9.5 percent.[6]

KNOW YOUR OMEGA NUMBERS

Measuring your red blood cell membrane level of omega fats may soon be a routine test as part of your blood lipid profile because the more we learn about the importance of these fats, these numbers may turn out to be as important, and possibly as predictive, as your blood cholesterol numbers. (See AskDrSears .com for the recommended omega-3 blood tests.)

In 2011–2012, I had the omega-3 index measured in fifteen patients in my medical practice to see if their red blood cell membrane levels correlated with the general dietary history of omega-3 intake. The graph shows that there is a reasonably good correlation. When I showed the low levels to some patients, they were motivated to eat more omega-3s. The lowest level, 3.3 percent, was in a 3-year-old boy who'd had multiple heart surgeries. I saw Michael in consultation because his parents wanted science-based nutritional advice to help heal his heart.

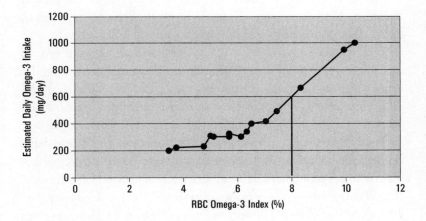

Fishy Burps

How can I get rid of that fishy burp taste after taking fish oil capsules?

Here are some ways to beat the burp: try enteric-coated fish oil capsules; get rid of the fishy taste by sucking on a lemon wedge after taking the capsules; take with food or orange juice; take the supplement right before bed. You may hear that freezing the capsules first reduces the fishy burp, but freezing can make them brittle and more prone to leak.

Plant Sources of Omega-3s

Is the omega-3 in flax oil as good as the omega-3 EPA/DHA from fish oil?

Flax oil is very healthy oil, and flaxseed meal (ground flaxseeds) is an excellent source of many phytonutrients. I enjoy 2 tablespoons of ground flaxseeds in my morning smoothie. Although flax oil is labeled an omega-3, it does not offer the same benefits in the body as omega-3 EPA/DHA from seafood. In the typical Western diet, even large doses of flax oil result in only small increases in the blood level of omega-3 EPA. Here's why.

The omega-3 in flax oil is called alpha linolenic acid (ALA) and it's a "short guy," only 18 carbon atoms long. Remember, the longer omega-3 carbon chains, such as EPA and DHA (20 and 22 carbon atoms long), work better in the body and brain. When you eat omega-3 EPA/DHA from seafood, it goes right to tissues, such as the brain and heart, where it's needed. DHA and EPA omegas are known as *preformed* omega-3 fatty acids, which means that no biochemical manipulation is needed by the body. The shorter omegas in flax oil, canola oil, and walnuts are *precursors*. When they are consumed, the liver must perform a series of complex biochemical steps called enzymatic processes to add two or four carbons to the "shorter guy" (ALA) chain to convert it into the "tall guy" EPA and DHA. The name of one of these enzymes is elongase, which makes the carbon chain longer. The body's efficiency in making this carbon add-on conversion varies from person to person. For some people, enzymes are picky converters and may not convert much of the flax oil omegas into EPA and DHA. They may convert less than 4 percent of the omega-3s in flax oil to DHA.[7] So if you take flax oil, do it *in addition to,* not instead of, fish oil.

Biochemists describe the conversion of ALA to EPA and

DHA as making the ALA molecules work uphill, and in some people these molecules are too lazy to do that. Best to eat the EPA/DHA molecules that are already at the top of the hill.

THE ESTROGEN EFFECT

The conversion of plant sources of omega-3, such as flax oil, may be slightly higher in premenopausal women than in men. Researchers have found that higher estrogen levels seem to slightly increase the conversion of the shorter-carbon precursors to DHA, a biochemical process called up-regulation.[8]

Omegas Added to Foods

Do omegas that have been added to foods offer the same health benefits?

Buyer beware! Now that omega-3s have gotten so popular, food packagers want to put them on their labels. Some will try to slip in some of the shorter, cheaper omega-3s, like those found in flax oil and canola oil, yet the package will still say "fortified with omega-3s." Here's a clue. If the label only says "omega-3s" it's probably from sources such as canola oil or flax oil and sometimes will say "omega-3 ALA." Look for labels that say "omega-3 DHA," "omega-3 EPA/DHA," or "omega-3s from marine sources."

Vegan Diets

I'm a vegetarian, and some of my friends are strict vegans — they don't eat any animal products or fish. How do we get more omega-3s into our diets?

I believe one of the healthiest diets in the world is the *pesco-vegetarian* diet, meaning seafood plus vegetables. This is why the

Mediterranean diet, which emphasizes seafood and vegetables, is so healthy. Since the omega-3s in plant foods like flax are not always metabolized efficiently in the human body, I advise my vegetarian patients to take daily omega-3 EPA/DHA fish oil supplements. Strict vegans could take DHA made from algae oil and EPA made from yeast.

Yet, vegetarian supporters of flax oil do have a valid point that they can get enough omega-3 DHA from plant sources, especially if they don't eat excess omega-6 oils, which may compete with the conversion of ALA to DHA.

A quarter cup of flaxseeds contains about 3600 mg ALA. One tablespoon of flax oil contains about 6000 mg ALA. One ounce of walnuts contains 2600 mg ALA. That seems like a lot of omega-3s compared to 2000–3000 mg of omega-3s in 6 ounces of salmon. Suppose a 4 percent conversion rate of ALA to EPA/DHA. Two tablespoons of flax oil yields 12000 mg of ALA. At 4 percent conversion, it would yield about 500 mg of omega-3s. At 1 percent conversion, it would yield only 120 mg of omega-3s. One ounce of walnuts at 2600 mg × .04 = 100 mg of omega-3s.

I recently saw Alice, a 47-year-old nurse, in consultation for dietary counseling. As a long-time confirmed vegan, she insisted she was getting enough omega-3s from her daily tablespoon of ground flax seeds. She didn't want to take fish oil supplements. I had her omega-3 red blood cell index measured, and it was at 3.6 percent, well below the optimal level of 8 percent. Being a wise nurse, she agreed to faithfully take a daily dose of 300 mg DHA from an algae source. After three months her red blood cell index had risen to 5.7 percent, which convinced her to continue taking daily omega-3 supplements (1000 mg) in addition to her daily flax. Even though the conversion of flax oil to omega-3 EPA/DHA is higher in premenopausal women because of the estrogen effect, that was not enough. (See tests for measuring omega-3 levels, page 160.)

Krill Oil?

It seems that krill oil is becoming more popular. How is this oil different from the usual fish oil?

Krill, tiny shrimplike seafood, are one of the most abundant cold-water species that larger fish eat. The two major omega-3 fatty acids in krill oil are the same found in fish, EPA and DHA, but unlike fish oils, most of the omega-3s in krill oil occur in phospholipid form. The health benefits of this biochemical difference remain unclear. The human body can use omega-3s in any of the three biochemical forms: triglyceride, phospholipid, and ethyl ester. All three omega-3 forms are well absorbed if taken with food, yet there is very limited evidence that the phospholipid form may be more easily absorbed than the other two. This preliminary evidence suggests that the body needs fewer metabolic steps and less energy to digest, absorb, and distribute the omega-3 phospholipids. Also, krill oil contains a small amount of the healthy pink pigment astaxanthin (see health benefits, page 180). Recent studies show krill oil to be a potent anti-inflammatory in helping alleviate rheumatoid arthritis.[9] (For updates, see www.AskDrSears.com.)

Egg Omegas

Are eggs a good source of omega-3s?

Yes, some eggs are, but not nearly as good as seafood. Egg yolks, but not egg whites, do contain some DHA, around 25 mg of DHA per yolk. This represents about 10–20 percent of the usual recommended daily dose of omega-3 EPA/DHA. Since there are no omega-3s in egg whites, unless you have a rare genetic problem called familial hypercholesterolemia and have been advised by your doctor, forget those egg-white-only omelets and enjoy the whole egg. Try not to overcook eggs, as this can destroy much of the DHA in the yolk, though this precaution is uncertain. Following the American Heart Association approval of eggs, I tell most of my patients, "An egg a day is okay."

While traveling in Greece, I noticed that not only do Greek eggs taste better, their yolks are deep yellow, almost orange. Greek hens roam free, eating plants rich in omega-3, and they may be fed some fish meal. The standard nutritionally deprived American hen is fattened with cheap omega-3-deficient chicken feed, resulting in eggs with pale yolks. A study showed that the ratio of omega-6s to omega-3s in egg yolk was 1.3 to 1 in free-range chickens and 19.9 to 1 for commercially raised chickens, and the yolk of eggs from hens fed fish meal contained six times the amount of omega-3s than the yolks of U.S. supermarket eggs.[10] This is another example of we are not only what we eat but also what the animals we eat eat.

Time It Takes to Increase Omega-3 Blood Level

I'm really taking my health seriously. How long do I need to eat extra omega-3s to get up to a healthy level?

According to the cardiovascular researcher Dr. William Harris, it depends on your starting level. If you are at 4 percent omega-3 index (like most Americans), then to raise your omega-3 index to the optimal level of 8 percent (see blood test, page 160), you would need to eat about 1000 mg of EPA/DHA per day for twenty-four weeks, 2000 mg per day for twelve weeks, or 3000 mg per day for eight weeks.[11]

Alcoholism

Can omega-3s help with alcoholism?

Possibly. Besides getting into a program such as Alcoholics Anonymous, alcoholics should eat lots of omega-3s. Eating more omega-3s may alleviate the nerve tissue damage from drinking excess alcohol. Since alcohol damages the fatty tissue in the brain, it makes sense that taking omega-3s, an important brain fat, could slow down the deterioration of the nervous tissue from drinking excess alcohol, called alcohol-induced neuropathy. Studies at the National Institutes of Health reveal that alcohol decreases DHA in brain cell membranes.[12]

Dr. Artemis Simopoulos, one of the early pioneers in the medical uses of omega-3s, theorized that the depressive effects of alcohol may be due to the fact that alcohol leaches DHA out of the brain. Alcohol also disrupts the chemical messengers in the brain, which is thought to be one of the reasons for the hangover effect. In addition to the direct toxic effects of alcohol on brain tissue, alcoholics usually suffer from an overall nutrition-deficient diet.

Alcohol and smoking decrease tissue levels of DHA.
—*Joseph Hibbeln, MD, National Institutes of Health*

It's in the Genes

How does consuming more omega-3s affect our genes?

Omega-3 EPA/DHA affects how your genes operate and does healthful things for them. The new science of *nutrigenomics* examines the relation between food and genes. Genes have little quirks that can predispose us to certain diseases (diabetes, for example). Yet each of these genes has an on/off switch. Some foods turn on (express) this gene, and the person eventually gets diabetes; other foods can turn off (suppress) this genetic tendency, preventing diabetes. Along with lots of fruits and vegetables, omega-3s help turn off these genetic tendencies for certain diseases.

Another name for these on and off switches on genes is "signaling pathways of metabolic processes." Omega-3 EPA/DHA seems to influence these pathways by turning on the healthful gene expressions and turning off the unhealthful ones. This scientific field is in its infancy, so once it grows up, we'll know more about how omega-3s affect the genes.

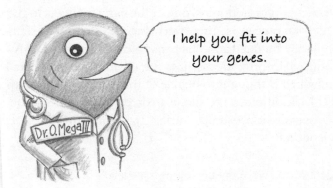

Quelling Cancer

Can omega-3s help prevent or alleviate cancer?

As a cancer survivor, I studied this question. What got me hooked on the value of omega-3s in my medical practice was the fact that the more omega-3 EPA/DHA you eat, the lower the incidence of the complications of just about every disease. Cancer is one of those diseases. While the scientific data are inconclusive, some studies suggest that the more omega-3s you eat, the less likely you are to get cancer:

- The EPIC (European Prospective Investigation into Cancer), one of the largest "eat more fish, lower your risk for cancer" studies, showed—after analyzing the dietary habits of thousands of people from ten European countries—that those who ate 10–20 ounces of fish per week were 30 percent less likely to get colon cancer.[13]

• A study in Scotland of nearly three thousand people showed that those who ate the most omega-3s had the lowest rate of colorectal cancer.[14]

• A 2006 Harvard study showed that men with the highest omega-3 to omega-6 blood ratios in their diets had the lowest risk of developing colorectal cancer.[15]

• A 2010 British study of people with precancerous colon polyps who took 2000 mg of omega-3 EPA daily for six months showed that the number and size of the polyps decreased, but the number and size of the polyps increased in the placebo-taking group.[16]

• A Swedish study of twenty-six hundred men showed that those who ate salmon more than once a week were 43 percent less likely to develop prostate cancer compared to men who ate none or ate salmon less frequently.[17]

• A Health Professionals Follow-up Study of forty-seven thousand men showed that those who ate more fish than others had a lower risk of developing prostate cancer.[18]

• A Swedish study showed that women who ate the most fatty fish had the lowest incidence of endometrial cancer.[19] Also, researchers have observed that people living along the coast who eat more fish suffer less colon cancer than city dwellers who eat less fish.

• Cancer specialists believe that because cancer patients tend to have low blood levels of omega-3s, eating more omega-3s may help these patients overcome the malnutrition that usually accompanies cancer and chemotherapy.[20]

The effect of omega-3 EPA/DHA in lowering cancer risk seems to be primarily on colon, prostate, and uterine cancers. Omega-3

EPA/DHA lowers cancer risk for several reasons. Researchers believe that omega-3s act like cell detoxifiers, yet excess omega-6s can act like cancer cell fertilizers. Again, omega balance is the key. A balance of omega-3s and omega-6s promotes healthy cell growth.

Back to the emerging science of nutrigenomics. Some of us are born with a family gene that increases our tendency to develop certain cancers. Yet, whether or not that gene is turned on and you get cancer, or turned off and you don't, can be influenced by certain nutrients, such as omega-3s. A cancer specialist described this as "omega-3s down-regulate the expression of the genes and also decrease the amount of proinflammatory chemicals, such as $COX2$ and prostaglandins, in the bloodstream that can fertilize the growth of cancer cells." In simple language, omega-3s turn down a dial on the genes that increase inflammation enough to cause cells to multiply out of control. Another possible mechanism of how omega-3s may reduce the risk of getting cancer is by increasing the self-destruction of cancer cells, a process called apoptosis.

Forgetting Your Fish Oil

I try to take my fish oil daily, but sometimes I forget. What should I do?

Because omega-3 EPA/DHA is a fat-soluble nutrient, it is stored in fat, so tissue levels remain reasonably constant, providing you continue a sufficient daily dose. This means if you miss a few days, you can continue your usual dose and your tissue omega-3 levels will soon build back up. Water-soluble nutrients, such as vitamin C, aren't stored this way, so you have to take them more often and the levels go down rapidly if you forget to take them. Yet omega-3 researchers caution that the body does not store omega-3s very long, which is why it's best to take them daily.[21]

Pet Protection

Should I be giving my pet fish oil?

Yes. Veterinarians have long appreciated the head-to-toe, or rather nose-to-tail, effects of adding omega-3s EPA/DHA to pet food. One of the most enlightening lectures on omega-3s I've ever attended was entitled "Protecting the Paws," in which the presenter gave an overview of all the healthful effects of omega-3s to improve the health of paws, skin and coat, eyes, joint mobility, and brain function.[22] The general conclusion was that omega-3s in pet food may be one of the reasons that pets are living longer, in addition to improved medical care. You should check with your vet about dosages of omega-3 supplements.

Too Much of a Good Thing

Can I eat too much fish oil?

While there is no official upper limit recommendation for a daily dose of omega-3s, the Food and Drug Administration recommends that people not take more than 3000 mg (3 grams) daily without a doctor's advice and supervision. Always discuss with your doctor what is the right dose for you. Eating this much in daily seafood would be highly unlikely—think 2½ pounds of oily seafood a day.[23]

Males Needing More

Do men need more omega-3s than do women?

Yes. Males seem to be affected more by omega-3 deficiencies than are females. The higher estrogen in females enables plant foods to be better converted into omega-3 EPA/DHA, and males tend to be more meat-eaters than plant-eaters. Females, just the opposite.

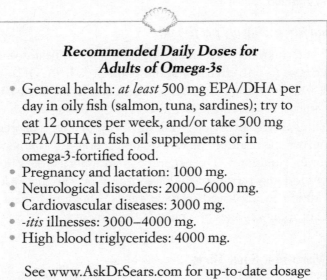

Recommended Daily Doses for Adults of Omega-3s

- General health: *at least* 500 mg EPA/DHA per day in oily fish (salmon, tuna, sardines); try to eat 12 ounces per week, and/or take 500 mg EPA/DHA in fish oil supplements or in omega-3-fortified food.
- Pregnancy and lactation: 1000 mg.
- Neurological disorders: 2000–6000 mg.
- Cardiovascular diseases: 3000 mg.
- *-itis* illnesses: 3000–4000 mg.
- High blood triglycerides: 4000 mg.

See www.AskDrSears.com for up-to-date dosage recommendations.

12

. . .

Selecting and Preparing Safe Seafood

Many of you suffer from seafood confusion: how much to eat and which seafoods are the safest and most nutritious. I want you to be wise seafood consumers, armed with the right questions to ask and knowing the right fish to pick. As I was undergoing my own lifesaving health makeover, the scientific fact that kept popping up was that people who eat more fish have healthier brains, hearts, joints, skin, blood, and a lower incidence of just about every ailment. Initially, I was not fond of seafood, but I was even less fond of getting sick. Here's my top health tip: "Go fish!"

When I polled my patients on the three main questions they had about selecting seafood, these were the most common questions:

- Which fish are the *safest* to eat?
- Which fish are the most *nutritious*?
- How much seafood should I eat weekly?
- Which fish are the tastiest and most *sustainable?*

Here's my step-by-step guide to selecting safe seafood.

EAT WILD!

You not only are what you eat, you are what the fish you eat eats. If the fish live in clean water and eat what fish are supposed to eat chances are they will be safe and nutritious to eat. Fish know what food is best for them better than fish farmers do.

Alaskan salmon is my favorite. All Alaskan seafood is grown in the wild. To continue sustainability, Alaska does have a hatchery program to augment their wild fisheries, but unlike farmed salmon, the baby salmon are released into the wild, where they grow up eating a wild diet and are subject to the same forces of nature that serve to cull the weak and sick. Nutritionally they are the same as those born in the wild. Since seafood is one of Alaska's top exports, authorities protect the fish with a proven fisheries management system that has become a model for the world.

Next time you're in a restaurant ordering seafood, "grill" the waiter: "Is the fish on your menu wild or farmed?" There is an unenforced regulation in the United States that seafood sellers must label fish "wild" or "farmed," but unfortunately farmed fish are sometimes sold as wild. When you see "Atlantic" on a menu, the fish is nearly always farmed. When you see "Alaskan" on a menu, it's always wild.

"But wild seafood is more expensive, and our family finances are tight. Is there that much difference?" a patient asked me.

I accepted the challenge: "What's your health worth? How much do you spend on prescription medicines per month?"

"Around fifty dollars," the patient said.

"How about those coffee latte treats?" I asked.

"About fifty dollars a month," the patient said.

"So that extra few dollars per pound for wild fish seems like a wise investment in your health. I suggest you spend that extra fifty dollars a month on a wild health insurance policy." As a general guide, wild salmon costs about $12–$14 more per pound than farmed. Note, most canned salmon is wild, and available year-round.

Fishing for Safe Seafood

My search for the safest seafood took me fishing in the pristine waters of Alaska. My favorite fisherman, Randy Hartnell, owner of VitalChoice.com, invited Martha and me as guests to Alaska to literally get a taste of how the habits of wild salmon affect their health benefits to humans, which was affirmed right after our first catch-and-cook meal. I call Alaskan fish "clean and lean" because they are relatively free of toxins and pollutants and are also lean on the extra omega-6 fats we don't need.

What a contrast with salmon raised in a fish farm. Those slow-swimming farmed salmon glide around their assigned space and eat cheap food all day. Like kids in a crowded classroom during flu season, they are more likely to spread infection. So antibiotics are sometimes added to their diet to prevent disease spreading.

Not only is the health of wild fish proof of the saying "You are what you eat," but this same fact of nutritional life is true for wild game and feedlot beef. You eat sticky meat, you get sticky blood. When I began my own health program, I compared the nutritional profile of feedlot-fed beef, which sit around in a pen and

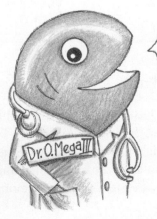

To get more vitamin D, enjoy sunshine and salmon.

eat junk food all day, to that of wild game like deer that run and graze on real food all day. The level of sticky stuff (unhealthy fats) is much higher in penned animals than it is in wild game. Since I love wild game (my hunter patients send me venison), I concluded that the same principles apply to wild fish.

I repeat, we are not only what we eat but what the animal we eat eats. When beef cattle went outside and played and grazed, beef contained some omega-3 oils. When food factories began to herd steers indoors to live in pens and eat junk food (grain-fed instead of wild plant–fed), the ratio of omega-3s to omega-6s reversed, as did the health of people in countries with a diet of less fish and more meat, and less range-fed and more feedlot-fed beef. Fortunately, consumer preference for grass-fed or range-fed meat is on the rise.

GO FISHING ONLINE

It's so easy to get safe, delicious frozen seafood and fish oil supplements online. (See Omega-3 Resources, page 204.)

A clever quote from a frequent online seafood selector:

Oh fish of the sea,
Swimming through cyberspace,
One click, you are mine.

— *Akiko Kobayashi*

Wild Fish Have a Healthier Omega Profile

Because wild fish eat natural fish food, they have a healthier omega-3 to omega-6 ratio in their meat than most farmed fish. The omega-6 content of farmed fish is higher, as is the case with any grain-fed livestock. For example, the levels of heart- and brain-healthy omega-3 fats, DHA and EPA, are higher in wild salmon.

Wild fish are lower in saturated fats. Farmed fish are generally fattier. When fish farmers took over from fishermen, the same downgrade happened to their product that happened in the beef industry. As beef builders fatten up their steaks, so do some fish farms.[1]

Wild Fish Are Higher in Vitamin D

A 2007 study by Boston University Medical Center researchers found that wild Pacific salmon had four times more vitamin D than farmed Atlantic salmon.[2] A 6-ounce serving of wild Alaskan sockeye salmon would give you about 1000 IU of vitamin D, which is the recommended minimum level per day. This study also showed that farmed salmon had three times as much fat as wild fish and a much greater proportion of omega-6 fats than omega-3s.

Wild Fish Are Naturally Pinker

Wild fish, such as salmon and mountain trout, contain more astaxanthin than farmed fish that are fed cheap food. The wild salmon get astaxanthin from krill, shrimp, and other marine life. Some farmed fish get their pink color from synthetic astaxanthin produced from petrochemicals in a laboratory, which may not be as biologically active.

EAT PINK!

The Healthy Color of Salmon

Why are salmon pink, you may wonder? My attraction to pink seafood began when in our sixties my wife and I took a dream vacation to climb the mountain of Machu Picchu in Peru. Before beginning our climb we were required to fill out a form revealing our age. We were pleasantly informed that we were the oldest people to climb the mountain that day. We were frequently passed by younger climbers who muttered, "Antiques," which I figured had something to do with old climbers.

During our mountain vacation we were treated to lake trout, also known as red salmon because of its reddish-pink color. Delving deeper into this delectable dish, I found out that the natives partly credit their health and longevity to this reddish-pink seafood. When we got back home, I had to do some "Pink Panther" detective work.

Let's follow my favorite color-changing fish, salmon, from ocean to spawning grounds, and you'll appreciate my prescription "Go fish!" even more. During the ocean phase of their life cycle, salmon feed on algae, krill, and small fish that are plentiful sources of astaxanthin. When the time comes for them to leave the ocean and, driven by some primitive GPS, return to their birth river to spawn and die, they will stop feeding, so they must depend upon the rich stores of fat, astaxanthin, and other nutrients they've accumulated at sea to sustain them during their final journey. The longer and more difficult this journey, the greater will be their stored energy reserves. In short, salmon returning to larger, longer, or more rapidly flowing rivers will generally provide the richest flesh.

To meet their energy needs, wild salmon store fat reserves required to sustain them after they leave the ocean. Because the good fat in wild salmon is so tasty and healthy, most are caught just before they leave the ocean, when their fat (and flavor) levels are at their peak.

Their flesh becomes pink by accumulating astaxanthin, which acts like a bodyguard to keep the fish muscle and fat strong and healthy. During their journey upriver, as the sockeye digest their stored fat, large amounts of astaxanthin migrate from their flesh into their skin, turning it bright crimson, hence their nickname, red salmon.

Strongly exercising muscles, like those in these fishy marathoners swimming upstream to mate, undergo oxidative stress, meaning lots of wear and tear. Astaxanthin blunts this muscle-fatiguing stress. Weight lifters and marathon runners often eat lots of antioxidants to help squelch oxidative stress.

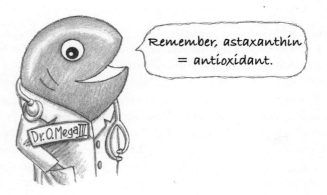

From Pink Fish to Human Athletes

Next, I wondered, where in the world do people eat like a salmon to compete in sports like a salmon? My next mission to learn more about this powerful pink antioxidant took me to the Big Island of Hawaii to the world's largest astaxanthin farm, where I spent the day with the nutritional researcher Bob Capelli.

Bob told me a fabulous fish story about how astaxanthin accumulates in the muscles of salmon and makes them the endurance heroes of the seafood world. This pink powerhouse preserves muscle strength and endurance in athletes (as it does in the salmon). It's a favorite nutritional supplement for Hawaiian seniors competing in Ironman Triathlons (swimming for 2 miles, then biking for 112 miles, capped by running for 26 miles). The local athletes dubbed astaxanthin "king of the carotenoids." (Carotenoids are a class of powerful antioxidants.)

BE YOUNG AND SMART—GO PINK!

Although the scientific data on astaxanthin are not yet conclusive, here's why we suspect astaxanthin is beneficial:

Astaxanthin benefits the brain. Dementia and many other brain Ds—OCD (obsessive-compulsive disorder), BPD (bipolar disorder), ASD (autism spectrum disorder)—are often associated with inflammation of the brain tissue. Simply speaking, sticky stuff accumulates in and around brain cells, keeping them from accurately communicating with each other. Astaxanthin can act like anti–sticky stuff medicine for the brain. Its unique biochemical structure enables it to cross the blood-brain barrier, the thin layer of tissue that acts like a protective wrap and prevents some chemicals from getting from blood to brain. Neurochemists call astaxanthin a *neuroprotectant* because of its ability to protect sensitive fatty brain tissue from oxidation. Astaxanthin is a powerful antioxidant, which simply means it prevents rust. Aging is like rusting.

Astaxanthin Benefits Vision. Remember, seafood is see food. Because the retina is actually part of the brain, what's good for the brain is also good for the eyes. The two top nutrients in the retina are omega-3s and carotenoids. Astaxanthin may be a more powerful antioxidant than the well-known carotenoids lutein and zeaxanthin. Carotenoids such as lutein and zeaxanthin are called nature's sunglasses because they protect the retina from sun damage and age-related macular degeneration. The retina is full of capillaries, those silver lining vessels. An interesting study showed that people taking astaxanthin had improved blood flow to their retina.[3]

How much astaxanthin should you eat? Because this colorful antioxidant is just beginning to be appreciated, there is not yet an official government Recommended Daily Intake (RDI) for astaxanthin. The average amount in salmon is around 6 mg astaxanthin per pound of salmon. (Wild sockeye salmon averages 20 mg per pound.) The usual supplement dose is 6 mg.[4] Many studies have used from 4 mg to 18 mg astaxanthin daily to get optimal health effects. For updated astaxanthin dosages, see www.AskDrSears.com.

FARMED FISH CAN ALSO BE HEALTH FOOD

Fish Are What They Eat

Eating farmed fish is certainly healthier than eating no fish. If fed nutritious fish food, farmed fish can actually be healthy for you. Farmed salmon fed pellets made from krill and fish meal can have omega-3 levels comparable to, or even higher than, wild salmon. However, those fed the less costly grain feed have less omega-3 and more omega-6 in their flesh. Admittedly, wild salmon may not always be plentiful enough to feed the world nor affordable for most people. For global sustainability, the healthiest solution is to regulate the fish-farming industry and enforce guidelines to help farmed fish approach the nutrient and environmental profile of wild fish. Right now there aren't adequate laws on how animals from the sea or land must be fed. If fish farms were required to feed their fish a diet close to the diet of wild fish, their product would be healthier, and our medical costs would likely go down.

It's shocking that we humans are feeding our farmed fish fake food. As a result, farmed fish have the same unhealthy fatty acid profile as some humans: too high in omega-6s and too low in omega-3s (an omega imbalance). For example, according to the

USDA nutrient database, farmed salmon has a healthy omega-3 to omega-6 ratio of 1:1, yet wild salmon enjoys a healthier ratio of 6:1 to 8:1. (See AskDrSears.com for updates on the fatty acid balance in various seafoods.)

Martha and I were working on this book one evening during dinner at a seafood restaurant. While taking our order, the waiter bragged about their "catch of the day," Kampachi, a local Hawaiian fish, being "high in omega-3s." This was the first time we ever heard that foodie promo, so we couldn't resist. After her first bite Martha smiled and said, "Hmm! This sure tastes fatty." Ordinarily, that would not be a heart-healthy observation when applied to a steak, but it was a compliment for seafood. After questioning the waiter, I learned this tasty fatty fish was actually farmed. I had to learn more.

My Visit to a Model Fish Farm

In recent years it has been fashionable to bash fish farming. So my quest to add some balance to "wild is best, but farmed is a close second" took me back to the Big Island of Hawaii to visit what is reputed to be a model fish farm, Kampachi Farms, where I visited with the marine biologist Neil Anthony Sims. Neil opened our conversation with, "If everyone in the world ate twelve ounces of seafood a week as you suggest, there would not be enough wild seafood to meet the demand. The amount of wild-caught fish has been flat for many years."

After he made the point that eating only wild seafood was possibly not sustainable to meet the growing demand, I asked Neil about the possible pollution problem of fish farming that some claim. He defended, "Aquaculture is greener than agriculture. It uses less fresh water, is more efficient at converting feed to sashimi, and doesn't produce the level of greenhouse gases that come from terrestrial livestock."

As a further defense of fish farming, Neil made a very important point that one of the ways to improve aquaculture and green farming is to take surplus food, such as land food, and develop ways of using this surplus land food to feed farmed seafood. That way you move away from the dependence on seafood and find a way to feed a nutritionally equivalent formula of land food to the farmed fish. That seems to be the goal of the green fish farmers.

The human body will live and grow on a less-than-nutritious diet. Not so for fish, who are much pickier eaters than humans. Farmed fish will not survive unless they have a reasonably nutritious diet, which contains enough seafood as fish meal to help them thrive. Neil calls this a market-driven approach: fish farmers want their fish to live and grow, which is why they use fish meal from omega-3-rich foods, such as anchovies and sardines, in addition to surplus oils from grains. He made the point that the best way to breed more fish is by retaining sustainability that is environmentally friendly and nutritionally equivalent. Neil likes to call this "softening your footprint on the sea."

Neil went on to give me a little lesson in fish feeding: "Fish eat proteins and fats. They don't eat carbs because marine fish are carbohydrate-intolerant. They can't digest starch. So the farmers extract the protein and oil from wheat and corn and put in the right balance of fatty acids from anchovies and fishing by-products, such as the guts, carcass, and bones, to make fish meal. As long as you get the right balance of protein and oil and omega-3s, the fish grow well." He showed me how they control the diet their fish eat "from hatch to harvest." There is a saying among fish farmers: "Bad food grows bad fish" (same as in human bodies), so I was interested in what food Neil feeds his fish.

Small fish are produced in the Kampachi hatchery and then released into a huge enclosed net pen a half mile offshore. Reputable fish farmers work to have a good feed-to-growth ratio, meaning how many pounds of feed it takes to grow 1 pound of fisา. At Kampachi it's about 1.6 pounds of feed to grow 1 pound of fish. Again, Neil made the point that they take from the surplus of the land and feed the deficiency of the sea. (My comment: Here is where wild seafood proponents would say, "Fish are supposed to eat fish food, not land food.")

Next our conversation went to "show me the science," particularly one of the themes of our book: the tissue is the issue. One of my concerns about farmed fish is that even though farmed fish can have the omega-3 content in their flesh equivalent to that of wild fish, the omega-6 content in the flesh of farmed fish is reputed to be much higher than that of wild fish. So I asked Neil what was the omega-6 to omega-3 ratio of his Kampachi fish. Neil showed me the data, which showed nearly a 1:1 ratio of omega-3s to omega-6s (specifically 970 mg of omega-3s to 860 mg of omega-6s per 1000 grams of flesh, and the EPA/DHA ratio was around 1:1). That convinced me that fish are really similar to humans: if fish eat the right food, their tissue will have sufficient omega-3s and omega-6s and in the right balance. Again, the ultimate way to improve fish farming is to make and enforce regulations on nutritional requirements for fish meal and to enclose the fish to keep their waste, disease, and parasites from escaping into the wild.

Will Wild Fish Last?

In his must-read book, *Four Fish: The Future of the Last Wild Food,* the fisherman and author Paul Greenberg writes that farmed fish may in fact be more polluted than wild fish with the remnants of old PCBs that are still bioconcentrated in the food chain. Wild salmon feed mainly on tiny shrimp and krill, which are very low in the food chain and therefore less likely to store PCBs. Farmed salmon, on the other hand, eat higher up in the food chain, small fish ground up for food, which tend to be higher in PCBs. Greenberg states that pollutants such as PCBs also accumulate in fatty tissue—farmed salmon average 15 percent fat content, whereas wild salmon average about 6 percent.

In the last twenty years, consumption of all salmon, farmed and wild, has doubled. According to Greenberg, one in three wild Alaskan salmon begins life in the hatchery. The hatchery process greatly increases the supply of wild salmon. The Alaskan Fish and Game managers claim that Alaskan hatchery supplementation is river-specific, meaning that the baby salmon are put back into the same river their parents came from, with the implication that they are genetically programmed to survive and thrive in that river. Also, in the wild about 80 percent of the eggs die before hatching. Yet, when raised in hatcheries, most will survive.

Wild salmon may be an enjoy-it-while-you-can scenario, since more people are craving wild salmon at a time when the world's salmon-supporting waterways are becoming fewer. As Paul Greenburg states, "We are eating into the principal of salmon stock instead of harvesting the annual interest." The conclusion then is that the supply will some time be bankrupt. Yet, I wish to add, from my conversations with Alaskan fishermen I have learned that because the salmon runs are sustainably managed and abundant, fishery managers ensure that only the "interest" is harvested.

EAT A VARIETY

Enjoy a variety of seafood, as each has its own nutritional perks. Some fish are higher in omega-3s; others are higher in vitamins and minerals. And each has its distinctive, delectable taste. Some fish lend themselves better to different preparations (grilling, sautéing, soups, patties, etc.). Give your gut a treat by enjoying as many of the green- and yellow-light species (see pages 186–187) as you can. Besides, some marine biologists believe that your risk of eating excess chemical pollutants is lower if you eat a variety of seafood.

EAT SAFE!

But what about mercury and other pollutants in seafood? In recent years many nutritionists, omega-3 researchers, and physicians have concluded that previous government seafood advisory warnings may have caused more harm than good, scaring consumers away from seafood. Let me emphasize that medical authorities who have thoroughly researched these guidelines, especially 12 ounces of any fish (except red-light ones) per week for everyone, conclude that except for red-light fish, the health benefits of seafood outweigh the risks.[5]

Since not everyone may be able to eat wild all the time, I distribute a handout in my medical office on selecting safe seafood, which classifies seafood by the green-yellow-red traffic-light method.

Traffic-Light Seafood Fishing[a]

Green-Light Fish	Yellow-Light Fish	Red-Light Fish
Safe, enjoy without limit.	Safe, enjoy up to 12 ounces per week.	Don't eat! Likely to be contaminated.
Anchovies	Bass, striped	King Mackerel
Artic char	Bluefish	Marlin
Butterfish	Carp	Shark
Catfish (U.S.)	Croaker, white, Pacific	Swordfish
Clams	Halibut, Atlantic	Tilefish, Gulf
Cod, Pacific	Lobster	of Mexico
Crab, Dungeness	Mahi-Mahi	
Crawfish	Monkfish	
Croaker, Atlantic	Orange roughy	
Flounder	Perch, freshwater	
Haddock, Atlantic	Rockfish	

Green-Light Fish	Yellow-Light Fish	Red-Light Fish
Safe, enjoy without limit.	Safe, enjoy up to 12 ounces per week.	Don't eat! Likely to be contaminated.
Hake	Sablefish	
Halibut, Alaskan	Sea bass, Chilean	
Herring	Shrimp, Atlantic	
Mackerel, North Atlantic	Skate	
Oysters	Snapper	
Perch, ocean	Tuna, albacore, yellow fin	
Pollock		
Rainbow trout		
Sablefish, Alaskan		
Salmon (canned, fresh, or frozen)		
Sardines		
Scallops		
Shrimp		
Sole		
Squid		
Tilapia		
Tuna, canned light		
Tuna, Pacific[b]		
Whitefish		
Whiting		

a. The seafoods listed here are categorized by mercury content. For the most up-to-date cautions about fish, visit www.AskDrSears.com. See the appendixes for related charts on the omega balance, nutritional content, and mercury levels of seafoods.

b. Know the source. Troll- and pole-caught tuna tend to be smaller and contain fewer contaminants than long-line, deep-water tuna, which tend to be larger and therefore more contaminated.

Source:
U.S. Department of Agriculture, "Dietary Guidelines for Americans," 2010.

SERVING SAFE FISH TO KIDS

Start serving seafood to children early, at around 8–9 months of age. (See how to shape young tastes, page 109.) Take extra safety precautions for kids. Children may be more vulnerable than adults to pollutants. The genetic machinery of rapidly dividing cells in growing tissue may be more affected by pollutants. Children's bodies have proportionally more fat than adults' bodies do. Brain tissue is 60 percent fat. Because pollutants are stored in fat tissue, they could be more dangerous to kids. Therefore, growing brains may be especially vulnerable to pollutants.

Here are guidelines that I teach in our medical practice and use for my family. Remember, these are just guidelines. Each family must make its own decision, especially if children have medical issues, such as any of the brain Ds.

- When possible, feed kids green-light seafood, about 12 ounces per week.
- Aim for the dosages recommended on page 153.

Over my years as a parent and child feeder, I've observed that busy moms don't like to count ounces. Anatomically, a child's fist is about the size of her tummy. When my kids were young, I used to compare their fist size with a serving size of salmon, and I came up with a rough guideline:

DR. BILL'S FISTFUL-OF-FISH RULE

Serve your child one fistful of safe seafood at least twice a week.

Cut a chunk of a seafood fillet the same size as your child's fist, and you'll be amazed how close it is to the 300–400 mg per day I recommend for young children. For example, a two-year-old's fist may equate in size to a 2–3-ounce salmon chunk. If eaten twice a week, that provides about 200–300 mg of omega-3 EPA/DHA per day. (As a general guide, wild salmon provides around 400 mg of omega-3 EPA/DHA per ounce.) (See page 153 for dosage guidelines for infants and toddlers.)

And if your child happens to be in a fish-loving mood, increase the offering that day. We all know those picky eaters may refuse it next week. Share my simple fistful-of-fish rule with your friends.

TEN TIPS ON GETTING KIDS TO EAT MORE SEAFOOD

Start Early. Begin serving tiny bits of salmon as one of your infant's earliest finger foods, at about 9 months of age. As has been proven in Asian cultures, babies who adapt to certain tastes enjoy them for a lifetime. This is called shaping young tastes.

Dip It. Children love to dip. Make yummy dips, such as hummus, teriyaki sauce, or marinara sauce, and let them dip pieces of salmon.

Sneak It. Mix seafood into their favorite recipes: fish tacos, spaghetti and salmon balls (instead of meatballs), burritos with strips of salmon, seafood soups, macaroni and cheese with chunks of salmon. Add drops of salmon oil or diced dried seaweed into your child's favorite foods. Put gradually increasing drops of fish oil into your child's favorite smoothie. Make fun fish dishes. Try salmon fish sticks, seafood teriyaki and fajitas, tuna wraps, and salmon quesadillas.

Cover It. If your child is not used to seafood, cover it with a favorite topping, such as cheese or homemade breading, or put

(continued)

the salmon under your child's favorite food, such as mashed potatoes or risotto rice on top. Hide the seafood under a proven favorite, such as cheese, pasta, tomato sauce, or mashed potatoes.

Sprinkle It. Sprinkle on their favorite topping that makes seafood tasty and enticing. Sprinkle on lemon or lime juice.

Spice It. Sprinkle on healthy spices that get your child's tastes used to these healthy condiments and help mask a fishy flavor: dill, fennel, lemon peel, garlic, turmeric, and pepper.

Sweeten It. Drizzle honey over a salmon fillet, and grill it to make a sweet glaze.

Share It. Use a little fishy peer pressure. Invite over some known seafood lovers and have a fish party. Your child is likely to want to copy his fish-loving friends.

Switch It. Instead of a beef burger serve a salmon burger. Just say, "We're having burgers tonight."

Prepare It Together. Children are more likely to eat what they help prepare in the kitchen.

Find recipes and seafood-fixing tips at www.AskDrSears.com.

SEAFOOD QUESTIONS YOU MAY HAVE

More Healthy Nutrients in Seafood

Besides omega fats, what other healthy nutrients are found in fish?

In addition to the healthy fats, namely, omega-3 EPA and DHA, there are many other healthful nutrients in fish, especially protein, vitamins D and B12, niacin, and selenium. These nutrients have a synergistic effect, meaning all the elements work together so that the whole health effect is greater than the sum of its parts. As an example of how Mother Nature protects her sea children, most seafood contains the mineral selenium, which acts like a mercury magnet to bind excess mercury and prevent it from reaching harmful levels.[6]

Cooking Questions

Does cooking fish destroy some of the omega-3s?

Seafood chefs who I consulted reassured me that the omega-3s in seafood are relatively resistant to heat. Yet, high heat could destroy some of the healthy fats and transform the omega fats into trans fats. With grilling, baking, steaming, and sautéing, the omega-3s are preserved.

FISH COOKING TIP

While grilling seafood on a fishing boat in Alaska, the chef taught me a cooking tip to preserve the flavor and texture of seafood: to avoid overcooking, remove the fish from the heat when it is 90 percent done. The heat from the flesh will naturally finish the remaining 10 percent.

Should I remove the skin from fish or eat it?

Fish skin is a good news and bad news situation. Some omega-3s are stored in the skin, so removing it removes some of the omega-3s. Yet, PCBs and other toxins are also stored in the skin and the fatty layer just beneath the skin. Eating these toxins can be minimized by removing the skin and surface fat. If your fish is from a safe source (e.g., wild Alaskan salmon), eat the skin. If you don't know, remove it.

Not Fond of Fish?

What if I really don't like fish?

Here's a story of how one of my patients, 42-year-old Paul, went from being a fish-hater to a fish-craver. Paul consulted me for a more nutraceutical way to treat his arthritis instead of taking so many pharmaceuticals. "I haven't eaten fish for forty-two years," Paul confided. "In fact, I hate fish!" Here's what the "fish doctor" prescribed: "Because the head brain and the gut brain (called the second brain) are connected, first convince your head brain how good seafood is for you. Next, eat a variety of safe sea-

---

IN SEARCH OF THE PERFECT FOOD

One evening after a nutrition talk, a guest asked me what I thought was the perfect food. I first considered that the perfect food would

* contain the most nutrients per calorie,
* contain the most important nutrients the body and brain need,
* be the most satisfying, or fill you up with less volume eaten,
* be tasty and nearly impossible to overeat,
* be just what the doctor ordered for the health of nearly every organ of the body.

All these clues led me to what I believe is the perfect food: a 6-ounce fillet of salmon, which contains more of the most vital nutrients per ounce than any other food I'm aware of. (See nutrient profile of salmon, Appendix C.)

---

food at least once a week and gradually build up to three times a week for three to six months." In addition, I asked Paul to take 2000 mg of fish oil daily. Within a month, Paul felt better. After two months, he said happily, "I not only wake up without joint pain, I actually crave fish!"

This taste reshaping is called metabolic reprogramming, in which the body learns to crave what it needs. I'm convinced there is a yet-to-be discovered "wisdom of the body" switch at the cellular level, perhaps in the gut lining, that acts as an inner voice, prompting us to "eat more of this, less of that." Turn on your inner seafood switch. After six months of eating my five S's diet: seafood, salads, smoothies, spices, and supplements, I craved these foods.

Sustainability

If we keep eating so much fish oil will the supply lessen?

This is a question that consumers naturally ask. I have gone to omega-3 conferences in which experts presented evidence saying that because only 3 percent of fish are used to produce fish oil, it's sustainable. Most of the omega-3 by-products of fishing are used for animal feed, and one-third of the fish caught are used for animal feed. The general consensus is that as long as there is global cooperation and oversight to improve and enforce sustainable aquaculture, humans will have enough fish to eat for a long time.

The good news is that rising concern about the health of our oceans and fisheries has led to increasing resources devoted to improving global fisheries management. As a result, many fish populations are recovering and stabilizing. The London-based Marine Stewardship Council (MSC) is considered by many to be the "gold standard" among a growing number of seafood sustainability organizations. You can do your part by choosing seafood from MSC-certified fisheries.[7]

MORE FOR LESS

A National Institutes of Health expert panel proposed a novel science-based "oil change" to help seafood sustainability. Since the tissue level of omega-3s is the target, if we ate less tissue-enzyme-competing omega-6 oil (e.g., corn oil, soy oil), we could achieve a healthy omega-3 effect even by eating less seafood.[8]

My Personal Diet

Dr. Sears, what diet are you on?

I think of the word *diet* as a positive term, meaning a way of eating, rather than as a restrictive word for what you can't eat. Most of my diet comprises these foods and ways of eating:

- I eat a real food diet, mostly off the land and sea.
- I mainly eat a five S's diet: seafood, salads, smoothies, spices, and supplements. These foods enjoy *synergy* (page 159).
- To keep my blood sugar stable, I graze by practicing my rule of 2s: eat twice as often, half as much, and chew twice as long. I not only eat fewer carbohydrates but partner them with protein, fiber, and fat, which steadies the absorption of carbs so that I don't get blood sugar highs and lows. And I "white out" dietary carbs by cutting way back on white bread, white pasta, and white pastries.
- On an average of five days a week I eat according to what I call the sipping solution. In the morning I make a full blender (64 ounces) of smoothie (see recipe at www .AskDrSears.com) and sip on this satisfying and delicious

drink all day long. It's my breakfast, lunch, and snacks. Then for dinner about four days a week I have seafood (usually salmon, tuna, halibut, or shrimp) and a hearty green salad on which I sprinkle turmeric and black pepper, garlic, and occasionally Indian spices like curcumin and ginger. The salad is so satisfying that it keeps me from overeating the rest of the meal. Eat green, stay lean!

- I begin each day with a high-protein breakfast.
- I often enjoy venison, a gift of wild game from my hunter friends.
- I eat a soft-boiled egg before bedtime a few nights a week.
- I nibble on nuts for extra energy on high-exercise days.
- I take a daily supplement of concentrated fruit and vegetable powder in capsule form, called Juice Plus.

After fourteen years of being on this diet, I'm enjoying a perfect blood chemistry profile: I am leaner, and my waist is 5 inches smaller than it was fifteen years ago. I enjoy what most seniors desire: Everything works and nothing hurts. What diet should you do? The one that works for you.

Safe Seafood Summary
- Top medical authorities conclude that the proven health benefits of seafood outweigh its possible risks.
- In selecting seafood,
  1. Ask where the fish grew up (place of origin). If it's Alaska, eat without worry. If not, then
  2. Check the seafood safety ranking in the table on pages 186–187. Except for "red light, don't eat" seafood, it is safe and advisable to eat 12 ounces per week of seafood even if you are pregnant or breast-feeding.
- To get the maximum nutritional benefits, eat a variety of seafood.
- For updates on safe seafood, visit www .AskDrSears.com.

Appendix A:
What Science Says about Omega-3 EPA/DHA's Healthful Effects

. . .

I wish there were a credit rating for scientific articles. In consultation with omega-3 experts I've attempted to separate those studies with an AAA rating (solid) from those in which the science is soft. While some science is solid and some is soft, there isn't another nutrient that offers so many of these health effects. This rating may change as research continues. Science says that omega-3 EPA/DHA

- protects brain, central nervous system, and cardiovascular system (solid);
- improves cognition (solid);
- controls inflammation (solid);
- is found in every cell of the body (solid);
- lessens autoimmune disorders (solid);
- reduces prostate cancer (solid);
- reduces fatal and nonfatal heart attacks (solid);
- reduces sudden cardiac death (solid);
- reduces stroke (solid);
- reduces atherosclerosis (solid);
- reduces triglycerides (solid);
- improves rheumatoid arthritis (solid);
- reduces age-related macular degeneration (solid);

- reduces symptoms of mood disorders, such as depression (solid);
- improves wound healing and nerve tissue injuries (solid);
- regulates immune response (soft);
- improves bone density (soft);
- delays the onset and lessens symptoms of Alzheimer's and dementia (soft);
- reduces the risk of certain cancers (soft);
- improves chronic fatigue syndrome (soft);
- lowers colorectal cancers (soft);
- reduces asthma (soft);
- reduces Crohn's disease and ulcerative colitis (soft);
- reduces schizophrenia (soft);
- reduces aggression (soft);
- reduces hearing loss (soft).

Many thanks to my Norway fishing friend and trusted omega-3 researcher, Dr. Jørn Dyerberg, for sharing with me his personal file of the most credible scientific articles. The science of the health benefits of omega-3 EPA/DHA evolves; see updates at www.AskDrSears.com.

Appendix B:
Helpful Chart for Selecting Safe Seafood

∗ ∗ ∗

Estimated EPA/DHA and Mercury Content in 4 Ounces
of Selected Seafoods

Common Seafoods	EPA/DHA mg/ 4 ounces[a,b]	Mercury mcg/ 4 ounces[c,d]
Salmon:[+] Atlantic,[*] Chinook,[*] Coho[*]	1200–2400	2
Anchovies,[*+] Herring,[*+] Shad[+]	2300–2400	5–10
Mackerel: Atlantic, Pacific (not King)	1350–2100	8–13
Tuna: Bluefin,[*+] Albacore[+]	1700	54–58
Sardines:[+] Atlantic,[*] Pacific[*]	1100–1600	2
Oysters: Pacific[e,f]	1550	2
Trout: Freshwater	1000–1100	11
Tuna: White (Albacore), canned	1000	40
Mussels:[+,f] Blue[*]	900	NA

(continued)

Common Seafoods	EPA/DHA mg/ 4 ounces[a,b]	Mercury mcg/ 4 ounces[c,d]
Salmon:[+] Pink,[*] Sockeye[*]	700–900	2
Squid	750	11
Pollock:[+] Atlantic,[*] Walleye[*]	600	6
Crab:[f] Blue,[+] King,[*+] Snow,[+] Queen,[*] Dungeness[*]	200–550	9
Tuna: Skipjack, Yellowfin	150–350	31–49
Flounder,[*+] Plaice,[+] Sole[*+] (Flatfish)	350	7
Clams[f]	200–300	0
Tuna: Light, canned	150–300	13
Catfish	100–250	7
Cod:[+] Atlantic,[*] Pacific[*]	200	14
Scallops:[+,f] Bay,[*] Sea[*]	200	8
Haddock,[*+] Hake[+]	200	2–5
Lobsters:[f,g] Northern,[*+] American[+]	200	47
Crayfish[f]	200	5
Tilapia	150	2
Shrimp[f]	100	0

Seafoods That Should Not Be Consumed by Women Who Are Pregnant or Breast-Feeding[h]

Shark	1250	151
Tilefish:[*] Gulf of Mexico[+,i]	1000	219

Common Seafoods	EPA/DHA mg/ 4 ounces[a,b]	Mercury mcg/ 4 ounces[c,d]
Swordfish	1000	147
Mackerel: King	450	110

* Seafood is included in EPA/DHA value(s) reported.

+ Seafood is included in mercury value(s) reported.

a. A total of 1750 mg of eicosapentaenoic (EPA) and docosahexaenoic (DHA) per week represents an average of 250 mg per day, which is the goal amount to achieve at the recommended 8 ounces of seafood per week for the general public.

b. EPA and DHA values are for cooked, edible portion rounded to the nearest 50 mg. Ranges are provided when values are comparable. Values are estimates.

c. A total of 39 mcg of mercury per week would reach the EPA reference dose limit (0.1 mcg/kg/d) for a woman who is pregnant or breast-feeding and who weighs 124 pounds (56 kg).

d. Mercury was measured as total mercury and/or methyl mercury. Mercury values of zero were below the level of detection. NA = data not available. Values for mercury adjusted to reflect 4-ounce weight after cooking, assuming 25 percent moisture loss. Canned varieties not adjusted; mercury values gathered from cooked forms. Values are rounded to the nearest whole number. Ranges are provided when values are comparable. Values are estimates.

e. Eastern oysters have approximately 500–550 mg of EPA/DHA per 4 ounces.

f. Cooked by moist heat.

g. Spiny lobster has approximately 550 mg of EPA/DHA and 14 mcg mercury per 4 ounces.

h. Women who are pregnant or breast-feeding should also limit white (albacore) tuna to 6 ounces per week.

i. Values are for tilefish from the Gulf of Mexico; does not include Atlantic tilefish, which have approximately 22 mcg of mercury per 4 ounces.

Sources:

U.S. Department of Agriculture, Agricultural Research Service, Nutrient Data Laboratory, 2011, USDA National Nutrient Database for Standard Reference, Release 24. Available at http://www.ars.usda.gov/ba/bhnrc/ndl.

U.S. Food and Drug Administration, "Mercury Levels in Commercial Fish and Shellfish (1990–2010)." Available at http://www.fda.gov/food/foodsafety/product-specificinformation/seafood/foodbornepathogenscontaminants/methylmercury/ucm115644.htm.

National Marine Fisheries Service, "National Marine Fisheries Service Survey of Trace Elements in the Fishery Resource." Report, 1978.

Environmental Protection Agency, "The Occurrence of Mercury in the Fishery Resources of the Gulf of Mexico." Report, 2000.

Appendix C
Average Nutrient Profile of Salmon

. . .

Nutrient Profile of 6 Ounces (170 grams) of Sockeye Salmon, Cooked, Dry Heat

		Percent Daily Value[a]
Calories	287	—
Protein	43 g	86[b]
Carbohydrate	0 g	0
Total fat	11 g	17
Omega-3 DHA	1200 mg[c]	—
Omega-3 EPA	1000 mg	—
Cholesterol	100 mg	33
Minerals		
Calcium	20 mg	2
Iron	0.85 mg	5
Magnesium	61 mg	15
Potassium	694 mg	20
Sodium	112 mg	5
Zinc	0.85 mg	6
Selenium	62 mcg	89

	Percent Daily Value[a]	
Vitamins		
Vitamin C	0 mg	0
Thiamine	0.37 mg	25
Riboflavin	0.24 mg	14
Niacin	16.5 mg	83
Pantothenic acid	2.33 mg	23
Vitamin B6	1.18 mg	59
Folate, total	15 mcg	4
Choline, total	191.6 mg	35
Vitamin B12	9.64 mcg	161
Vitamin A	352 IU	7
Vitamin E	1.94 mg	10
Vitamin D	894 IU	224[d]
Astaxanthin	8 mg	—[e]

g = grams; mg = milligrams; mcg = micrograms; IU = international units.

a. Percent Daily Values are based on a 2000-calorie per day diet.

b. This is the USDA Daily Value for protein, but I believe most adults need around 0.75 grams of protein per pound of their ideal body weight.

c. There is a wide range of omega-3 EPA/DHA content in seafood, depending on the species, time of year, and processing. While an official Daily Value for omega-3 EPA/DHA has yet to be released by the USDA, 500–1000 mg per day is the general recommendation by most authorities.

d. Percent Daily Value of vitamin D is in the process of being revised upward.

e. See astaxanthin effects, page 181.

Source:
USDA National Nutrient Database for Standard Reference, 2011.

Omega-3 Resources

. . .

Books

William Lands. *Fish, Omega-3 and Human Health.* 2d ed. AOCS Books, 2005.

Joseph C. Maroon and Jeffrey Bost. *Fish Oil: The Natural Anti-inflammatory.* Basic Health Publications, 2006.

Web Resources

www.AskDrSears.com. For updates to *The Omega-3 Effect* and our top selections of omega-3 fish oil supplements and seafoods.

www.VitalChoice.com. Publishes *Vital Choices,* a twice-weekly newsletter with nuggets of easy-to-read information on new omega-3 fish oil research.

www.FatsofLife.com. Publishes *Fats of Life Newsletter,* quarterly newsletter on past and present omega-3 research on heart health, pregnancy and infancy, mental health, behavioral disorders, and other health concerns.

www.GOEDomega3.com. Global Organization for EPA and DHA Omega-3, an association of omega-3 EPA and DHA supporters working to educate consumers and the health care industry on the health benefits of omega-3 EPA/DHA. A rich source of scientific information on the health benefits of fish oil.

Safe and Sustainable Seafood Sources

www.VitalChoice.com. Our top choice for wild Pacific seafood, organic food selections, and gift packages.

www.MSC.org. Marine Stewardship Council, a prominent seafood sustainability organization. Many trusted seafood companies display the MSC seal for certified sustainable seafood.

www.MontereyBayAquarium.org. Obtain a Seafood Watch pocket card of green-, yellow-, and red-light seafood. The Seafood Watch app for mobile phones gives markets and restaurants that have sustainable seafood.

Blood Test Kits for Measuring Omega Levels

www.OmegaQuant.com.

www.VitalTest.com.

Acknowledgments

. . .

Besides the scientific experts introduced on pages xi–xii, other members of the omega-3 team whom I wish to thank are Randy Hartnell, owner of Vital Choice Seafood Company, for teaching me about selecting safe seafood; the omega-3 researcher Dr. Eric Lien for his critique of the manuscript; many patients in my medical practice who gave me a consumer critique of this book, prompting me to keep it simple and make it fun to read; Tracee Zeni, my assistant and tireless typist for twenty-one years; and Tracy Behar, Christina Rodriguez, Peggy Freudenthal, Karen Landry, and Alice Cheyer for their reader-friendly advice.

Notes

• • •

Chapter 1 Four Fish Stories

1. W. H. Oddy, L. Jianghong, A. J. Whitehouse et al., Breastfeeding duration and academic achievement at 10 years, *Pediatrics* 127 (2011): e137–e145.
2. Read about my personal story from sickness to health, and the head-to-toe wellness plan I developed, in my book *Prime-Time Health: A Scientifically Proven Plan for Feeling Young and Living Longer* (Little, Brown, 2010).
3. H. O. Bang, J. Dyerberg, and A. B. Nielsen, Plasma lipid and lipoprotein pattern in Greenlandic West-Coast Eskimos, *Lancet* 297 (June 5, 1971): 1143–1146; J. Dyerberg and H. O. Bang, Haemostatic function and platelet polyunsaturated fatty acids in Eskimos, *Lancet* 314 (Sept. 1, 1979): 433–435; H. O. Bang, J. Dyerberg, and H. M. Sinclair, The composition of the Eskimo food in north western Greenland, *American Journal of Clinical Nutrition* 33 (Dec. 1980): 2657–2661.
4. In a personal communication in March 2011, Dr. Dyerberg provided these details of his study results:

	Inuits	Danes
Fats in diet		
Saturated (%)	22.0	52.0
Omega-3s (grams/day)	13.7	2.8
Omega-6s (grams/day)	5.4	10.0
Omega-3/Omega-6 ratio	2.5	0.3
Blood tests		
Bleeding times (minutes)	8.1	4.7
Omegas in blood platelets		
Omega-6 (AA) (%)	8.5	22.0
Omega-3 (EPA) (%)	8.0	0.5

Chapter 2 What Are Omega-3s, and Why Are They So Healthy?

1. *The Doctor Oz Show*, "The Big O: Know Your Omegas," January 26, 2011, and April 1, 2011. You may see omegas identified with numbers in medical articles: 18:3n-3 (ALA), 20:5n-3 (EPA), 18:2n-6 (LA); 20:4n-6 (AA); 22:6n-3 (DHA). For example, for DHA, 22 means number of carbon atoms, 6n means number of double bonds, and -3 means first double bond in third position from the end.

2. Nutritional Armor for the Warfighter: Can Omega-3 Fatty Acids Enhance Resilience, Wellness, and Military Performance? Conference at the National Institutes of Health, October 13, 2009. This seven-hour videocast is a must-view to see the Top Docs present the top science of omega-3s. Available at http://videocast.nih.gov/summary.asp?live=8107.

3. For more information on omega balance biochemistry and why the tissue is the issue, see Fats and fatty acids in human nutrition: Report of an expert consultation, *WHO*, 2008, http://www.fao.org/docrep/013/i1953e/i1953e00.pdf.

4. W. E. Lands, *Fish, Omega-3 and Human Health*, 2d ed. (AOCS Books, 2005); J. R. Hibbeln, L. Nieminen, T. L. Blasbalg et al., Healthy intakes of n-3 and n-6 fatty acids: Estimations considering worldwide diversity, *American Journal of Clinical Nutrition* 83 (2006): S1483–S1493; L. G. Cleland, M. J. James, M. A. Neumann et al., Linoleate inhibits EPA incorporation from dietary fish-oil supplements in human subjects, *American Journal of Clinical Nutrition* 55 (1992): 395–399; C. E. Ramsden, J. R. Hibbeln, S. F. Majchrzak et al., n-6 fatty acid-specific and mixed polyunsaturate dietary interventions have different effects on CHD risk: A meta-analysis of randomised controlled trials, *British Journal of Nutrition* 104 (2010): 1586–1600; L. M. Arterburn, E. B. Hall, and H. Oken, Distribution, interconversion, and dose response of n-3 fatty acids in humans, *American Journal of Clinical Nutrition* 83 (2006): S1467–S1476; T. L. Blasbalg, J. R. Hibbeln, C. E. Ramsden et al., Changes in consumption of omega-3 and omega-6 fatty acids in the United States during the twentieth century, *American Journal of Clinical Nutrition* 93 (2011): 950–962.

The authors of the last article studied how omega-6 in the Western diet has markedly increased from 1909 to 1999. They found that
- the per capita consumption of soybean oil increased more than a thousandfold over the past hundred years;

- the ratio of dietary omega-6s to omega-3s increased from 1:1 to as much as 30:1 in the standard American diet over the past decade;
- the omega-6–LA (linoleic acid) content of breast milk in U.S. women doubled from 1945 to 1965, from 6–7 percent to 15–16 percent of total fatty acids;
- the omega-6–LA content of fat tissue increased from 6 percent in 1960 to 18 percent in 1986.

5. D. Mozaffarian, A. Ascherio, F. B. Hu et al., Interplay between different polyunsaturated fatty acids and risk of coronary heart disease in men, *Circulation* 111 (2005): 157–164; T. Pischon, S. E. Hankinson, G. S. Hotamisligil et al., Habitual dietary intake of n-3 and n-6 fatty acids in relation to inflammatory markers among U.S. men and women, *Circulation* 108 (2003): 155–160; W. S. Harris, The omega-6/omega-3 ratio and cardiovascular disease risk: Uses and abuses, *Current Atherosclerosis Reports* 8 (2006): 453–459; Omega-6 fatty acids and risk for cardiovascular disease: A science advisory from the American Heart Association Nutrition Subcommittee of the Council on Nutrition, Physical Activity, and Metabolism, Council on Cardiovascular Nursing, and Council on Epidemiology and Prevention, *Circulation* 119 (2009): 902–907.

The conclusion of some researchers is that the high dietary ratio of sticky fats (saturated and trans fats) to omega-3, but not the ratio of omega-6 to omega-3, seems to be a marker for coronary artery disease and inflammation.

6. A. M. Marina, Y. B. Che Man, and I. Amin. Virgin coconut oil: Emerging functional food oil, *Trends in Food Science and Technology* 20 (2009): 481–487.

7. W. S. Harris, Personal communication, April 2011.

Chapter 3 How Omega-3s Help Your Heart

1. G. Danaei, E. L. Ding, D. Mozaffarian et al., The preventable causes of death in the United States: Comparative risk assessment of dietary, lifestyle, and metabolic risk factors, *PLoS* 6 (2009).

2. W. S. Harris, K. J. Reid, S. A. Sands et al., Blood omega-3 and trans fatty acids in middle-aged acute coronary syndrome patients, *American Journal of Cardiology* 99 (2007): 154–158; S. Wang, A. Q. Ma, S. W. Song et al., Fish oil supplementation improves large arterial elasticity

in overweight hypertensive patients, *European Journal of Clinical Nutrition* 62 (2008): 1426–1431.

3 S. A. Wright, F. M. O'Prey, M. T. McHenry et al., A randomised placebo-controlled interventional trial of omega-3 polyunsaturated fatty acids on endothelial function and disease activity in systemic lupus erythematosus, *Annals of the Rheumatic Diseases* 67 (2008): 841–848; L. J. Ignarro, *No More Heart Disease* (St. Martin's Press, 2005); M. C. Houston, *Vascular Biology in Clinical Practice* (Hanley and Belfus, 2002).

4. P. Nestel, H. Shige, S. Pomeroy et al., The n-3 fatty acids eicosapentaenoic acid and docosahexaenoic acid increase systemic arterial compliance in humans, *American Journal of Clinical Nutrition* 76 (2002): 326–330.

5. N. M. de Roos, M. L. Bots, and M. B. Katan, Replacement of dietary saturated fatty acids by trans fatty acids lowers serum HDL cholesterol and impairs endothelial function in healthy men and women, *Arteriosclerosis, Thrombosis, and Vascular Biology* 21 (2001): 1233–1237.

6. W. S. Harris, K. J. Reid, S. A. Sands et al., Blood omega-3 and trans fatty acids in middle-aged acute coronary syndrome patients, *American Journal of Cardiology* 99 (2007): 154–158; A. F. Cicero, S. Ertek, and C. Borghi, Omega-3 polyunsaturated fatty acids: Their potential role in blood pressure prevention and management, *Current Vascular Pharmacology* 7 (2009): 330–337; M. P. Pase, N. A. Grima, and J. Sarris, The effects of dietary and nutrient interventions on arterial stiffness: A systematic review, *American Journal of Clinical Nutrition* 93 (2011): 446–454; S. Wang, A. Q. Ma, S. W. Song et al., Fish oil supplementation improves large arterial elasticity in overweight hypertensive patients, *European Journal of Clinical Nutrition* 62 (2008): 1426–1431; H. Ueshima, J. Stamler, P. Elliott et al., Food omega-3 fatty acid intake of individuals (total, linolenic acid, long-chain) and their blood pressure: INTERMAP study, *Hypertension* 50 (2007): 313–319.

7. J. N. Din, S. A. Harding, C. J. Valerio et al., Dietary intervention with oil rich fish reduces platelet-monocyte aggregation in man, *Atherosclerosis* 197 (2008): 290–296.

8. T. Huang, J. Zheng, Y. Chen et al., High consumption of omega-3 polyunsaturated fatty acids decreases plasma homocysteine: A meta-analysis of randomized, placebo-controlled trials, *Nutrition* 27 (2011): 863–867.

9. M. Yokoyama, H. Origasa, M. Matsuzaki et al., Effects of eicosapentaenoic acid on major coronary events in hypercholesterolemic patients (JELIS): A randomised open-label, blinded endpoint analysis, *Lancet* 369 (Mar. 2007): 1090–1098.

10. Information about the long-running Physicians' Health Study is available at http://phs.bwh.harvard.edu.

11. T. Huang, J. Zheng, Y. Chen et al., High consumption of omega-3 polyunsaturated fatty acids decreases plasma homocysteine: A meta-analysis of randomized, placebo-controlled trials, *Nutrition* 27 (2011): 863–867.

12. This study found that giving 810 mg per day of omega-3 EPA/DHA to patients with coronary artery disease showed beneficial cardioprotective effects of decreasing resting heart rate, increasing postexercise heart rate recovery, and generally improving the overall sympathetic and vagus nerve monitoring of cardiac function. J. H. O'Keefe, H. Abuissa, A. Sastre et al., Effects of omega-3 fatty acids on resting heart rate, heart rate recovery after exercise, and heart rate variability in men with healed myocardial infarctions and depressed ejection fractions, *American Journal of Cardiology* 97 (2008): 1127–1130.

13. R. Marchioli, F. Barzi, E. Bomba et al., Early protection against sudden death by n-3 polyunsaturated fatty acids after myocardial infarction, *Circulation* 105 (2002): 1897–1903; C. M. Albert, H. Campos, M. J. Stampfer et al., Blood levels of long-chain n-3 fatty acids and the risk of sudden death, *New England Journal of Medicine* 346 (2002): 1113–1118; T. Amano, T. Matsubara, T. Uetani et al., Impact of omega-3 polyunsaturated fatty acids on coronary plaque instability, *Atherosclerosis* 218 (2011): 110–116; L. Calò, L. Bianconi, F. Colivicchi et al., n-3 fatty acids for the prevention of atrial fibrillation after coronary artery bypass surgery, *Journal of the American College of Cardiology* 45 (2005): 1723–1728.

The study described in the last article found that a dosage of 1700 mg per day of omega-3 EPA/DHA reduced the occurrence of atrial fibrillation by 54 percent after patients underwent coronary artery bypass surgery.

14. R. Marchioli, F. Barzi, E. Bomba et al., Dietary supplementation with n-3 polyunsaturated fatty acids and vitamin E after myocardial infarction: Results of the GISSI-Prevenzione trial, *Lancet* 354 (1999): 447–455.

Further analysis of the GISSI study data showed a 95 percent reduction in sudden cardiac death in persons supplemented with omega-3s. R. Marchioli, F. Barzi, E. Bomba et al., Early protection against sudden death by n-3 polyunsaturated fatty acids after myocardial infarction: Time-course analysis of the results of the GISSI-Prevenzione study, *Circulation* 105 (2002): 1897–1903.

15. H. C. McGill Jr., C. A. McMahan, and S. S. Gidding, Preventing heart disease in the 21st century: Implications of the pathobiological determinants of atherosclerosis in youth, *Circulation* 117 (2008): 1216–1227.

16. M. H. Pedersen, C. Mølgaard, L. I. Hellgren et al., Effects of fish oil supplementation on markers of the metabolic syndrome, *Journal of Pediatrics* 157 (2010): 395–400.

17. F. B. Hu, E. Cho, K. M. Rexrode et al., Fish and long-chain omega-3 fatty acid intake and risk of coronary heart disease and total mortality in diabetic women, *Circulation* 107 (2003): 1852–1857; F. B. Hu, L. Bronner, W. C. Willet et al., Fish and omega-3 fatty acid intake and risk of coronary heart disease in women, *JAMA* 287 (2002): 1815–1821.

18. S. G. West, Effect of diet on vascular reactivity: An emerging marker for vascular risk, *Current Atherosclerosis Reports* 3 (2001): 446–455.

19. H. M. Roche and M. J. Gibney, Effect of long-chain n-3 polyunsaturated fatty acids on fasting and postprandial triacylglycerol metabolism, *American Journal of Clinical Nutrition* 71 (2000): 232S–237S; M. D. Griffin, T. A. Sanders, I. G. Davies et al., Effects of altering the ratio of dietary n-6 to n-3 fatty acids on insulin sensitivity, lipoprotein size, and postprandial lipemia in men and postmenopausal women aged 45–70 y: The OPTILIP study, *American Journal of Clinical Nutrition* 84 (2005): 1290–1298.

20. Here's what scientists have said about omega-3s and bleeding concerns.

W. S. Harris, Expert opinion: Omega-3 fatty acids and bleeding — cause for concern? *American Journal of Cardiology* 99 (2007): 44C–46C; P. D. Watson, P. S. Joy, C. Nkonde et al., Comparison of bleeding complications with omega-3 fatty acids+aspirin+clopidogrel versus aspirin+clopidogrel in patients with cardiovascular disease, *American Journal of Cardiology* 104 (2009): 1052–1054.

I. K. Bender, M. A. Kraynak, E. Chiquette et al., Effects of marine fish oils on the anticoagulation status of patients receiving chronic warfarin therapy, *Journal of Thrombosis and Thrombolysis* 5 (1998):

257–261. In this study, patients who were already being treated with warfarin were given 3–6 grams of fish oil daily in addition to their current therapy. This was a double-blind, placebo-controlled, randomized study. The conclusion: There was no significant difference in measures of blood coagulation (INRs) between the placebo group and the treatment group. The authors also concluded that the benefits of taking fish oil to reduce clotting outweigh the risk, especially in people who are taking anticoagulants to avoid reclotting of previous coronary artery thrombosis.

Yet, a 2004 article reported a single case of a patient on warfarin therapy who was taking 1–2 grams of fish oil a day and showed an increase in INR from 2.8 to 4.3 within one month. One week after reducing the fish oil dose, the INR decreased to 1.6. The conclusion of some researchers was that omega-3 fatty acids in doses exceeding 3000–4000 mg (3–4 grams) per day are associated with a moderate increase in INR, which has led the Food and Drug Administration to issue a caution on doses over 3000 mg (3 grams) per day. M. S. Buckley, A. D. Goff, and W. E. Knapp, Fish oil interaction with warfarin, *Annals of Pharmacotherapy* 38 (2004): 50–52.

J. Eritsland, H. Arnesen, I. Seljeflot et al., Long-term effects of n-3 polyunsaturated fatty acids on haemostatic variables and bleeding episodes in patients with coronary artery disease, *Blood Coagulation and Fibrinolysis* 6 (1995): 17–22; T. G. Guilliams, The use of fish oil supplements in clinical practice: A review, *Journal of the American Nutraceutical Association* 8 (2005): 21–34; H. Iso, K. M. Rexrode, M. J. Stampfer et al., Intake of fish and omega-3 fatty acids and risk of stroke in women, *JAMA* 285 (2001): 304–312.

The Physicians' Health Study showed a lowered risk of stroke with increasing fish consumption in men. K. He, E. B. Rimm, A. Merchant et al., Fish consumption and risk of stroke in men, *JAMA* 288 (2002): 3130–3136.

Scientists who treated people with severe neurological disorders with 6 grams of omega-3 EPA/DHA daily did not notice dangerous bleeding tendencies in their patients. C. Wang, W. H. Harris, M. Chung et al., n-3 fatty acids from fish or fish-oil supplements, but not alpha-linolenic acid, benefit cardiovascular disease outcomes in primary- and secondary-prevention studies: A systematic review, *American Journal of Clinical Nutrition* 84 (2006): 5–17.

J. Eritslend, Safety considerations of polyunsaturated fatty acids, *American Journal of Clinical Nutrition* 71 (2000): S197–S201; H. R. Knapp, Dietary fatty acids in human thrombosis and hemostasis, *American Journal of Clinical Nutrition* 65 (1997): S1687–S1698.

21. M. Yokoyama, H. Origasa, M. Matsuzaki et al., Effects of eicosapentaenoic acid on major coronary events in hypercholesterolemic patients (JELIS): A randomised open-label, blinded endpoint analysis, *Lancet* 369 (Mar. 2007): 1090–1098.

22. GISSI-HF investigators. Effect of n-3 polyunsaturated fatty acids in patients with chronic heart failure (the GISSI-HF trial): A randomised, double-blind, placebo-controlled trial, *Lancet* 372 (2008): 1223–1230.

23. R. Marchioli, F. Barzi, E. Bomba et al., Early protection against sudden death by n-3 polyunsaturated fatty acids after myocardial infarction. *Circulation* 105 (2002): 1897–1903; F. B. Hu, E. Cho, K. M. Rexrode et al., Fish and long-chain omega-3 fatty acid intake and risk of coronary heart disease and total mortality in diabetic women, *Circulation* 107 (2003): 1852–1857; W. Davis, New blood test better predicts heart attack risk, *Life Extension Magazine*, May 2006.

Chapter 4 How Omega-3s Build Smarter Brains and Better Moods

1. J. T. Brenna, Personal communication, December 2011.

2. R. L. Aupperle, D. R. Denney, S. G. Lynch et al., Omega-3 fatty acids and multiple sclerosis: Relationship to depression, *Journal of Behavioral Medicine* 31 (2008): 127–135; L. Shinto, G. Marracci, S. Baldauf-Wagner et al., Omega-3 fatty acid supplementation decreases matrix metalloproteinase-9 production in relapsing-remitting multiple sclerosis, *Prostaglandins Leukotrienes and Essential Fatty Acids* 80 (2009): 131–136; B. Weinstock-Guttman, M. Baier, Y. Park et al., Low fat dietary intervention with omega-3 fatty acid supplementation in multiple sclerosis patients, *Prostaglandins Leukotrienes and Essential Fatty Acids* 73 (2005): 397–404.

3. G. Bartzokis, Personal communication, June 2011.

4. G. Bartzokis, Neuroglialpharmacology: White matter and psychiatric treatments. *Frontiers in Bioscience* 17 (2011): 2695–2733.

5. B. K. Puri, G. M. Bydder, M. S. Manku et al., Reduction in cerebral atrophy associated with ethyl-eicosapentaenoic acid treatment in patients with Huntington's disease, *Journal of International Medical Research* 36 (2008): 896–905.

6. J. P. Infante, R. C. Kirwan, and J. T. Brenna, High levels of doccsa-hexaenoic acid (22:6n-3)-containing phospholipids in high-frequency contraction muscles of hummingbirds and rattlesnakes, *Comparative Biochemistry and Physiology Part B* 130 (2001): 291–298.

7. C. L. Broadhurst, S. C. Cunnane, and M. A. Crawford, Rift Valley lake fish and shellfish provided brain-specific nutrition for early Homo, *British Journal of Nutrition* 79 (1998): 3–21.

8. E. J Johnson, H. Y. Chung, S. M. Caldarella et al., The influence of supplemental lutein and docosahexaenoic acid on serum, lipopro-teins, and macular pigmentation, *American Journal of Clinical Nutrition* 87 (2008): 1521–1529.

9. C. Williams, E. E Birch, P. M. Emmett et al., Stereoacuity at age 3.5 y in children born full-term is associated with prenatal and postnatal dietary factors, *American Journal of Clinical Nutrition* 73 (2001): 316–322.

10. M. Roncone, H. Bartlett, and F. Eperjesi, Essential fatty acids for dry eye: A review, *Contact Lens and Anterior Eye* 33 (2010): 49–54; J. C. Wojtowicz, I. Butovich, E. Uchiyama et al., Pilot, prospective, ran-domized, double-masked, placebo-controlled clinical trial of an omega-3 supplement for dry eye, *Cornea* 30 (2011): 308–314.

11. J. P. SanGiovanni, E. Y. Chew, T. E. Clemons et al., The relationship of dietary lipid intake and age-related macular degeneration in a case-control study: AREDS report 20, *Archives of Ophthalmology* 125 (2007): 671–679; W. G. Christen, D. A. Schaumberg, R. J. Glynn et al., Dietary omega-3 fatty acid and fish intake and incident age-related macular degeneration in women, *Archives of Ophthalmology* 129 (2011): 921–929; J. S. Tan, J. J. Wang, V. Flood et al., Dietary fatty acids and the ten-year incidence of age-related macular degeneration: The Blue Mountains eye study, *Archives of Ophthalmology* 127 (2009): 656–665; J. P. Sangiovanni, E. Agrón, A. D. Meleth et al., Omega-3 long-chain polyunsaturated fatty acid intake and 12–y incidence of neovascular age-related macular degeneration and central geographic atrophy: AREDS report 30, *American Journal of Clinical Nutrition* 90 (2009): 1601–1607.

12. M. Peet and C. Stokes., Omega-3 fatty acids in the treatment of psy-chiatric disorders, *Drugs* 65 (2005): 1051–1059; M. Maes, A. Chris-tophe, J. Delanghe et al., Lowered omega-3 polyunsaturated fatty acids in serum phospholipids and cholesteryl esters of depressed patients, *Psychiatry Research* 85 (1999): 275–291; T. McCarren, R.

Hitzemann, R. Smith et al., Amelioration of severe migraine by fish oil (omega-3) fatty acids, *American Journal of Clinical Nutrition* 41 (1985): 874 (abstract); M. Peet and D. F. Horrobin, A dose-ranging study of the effects of ethyl-eicosapentaenoate in patients with ongoing depression despite apparently adequate treatment with standard drugs, *Archives of General Psychiatry* 59 (2002): 913–919.

Summarizing these scientific studies, the general conclusion was that EPA alone or in combination with DHA improves mood disorders, whereas DHA supplementation only does not. P. Y. Lin and K. P. Su, A meta-analytic review of double-blind, placebo-controlled trials of antidepressant efficacy of omega-3 fatty acids, *Journal of Clinical Psychiatry* 68 (2007): 1056–1061. See also F. L. Crowe, M. Skeaff, T. J. Green et al., Serum phospholipid n-3 long-chain polyunsaturated fatty acids and physical and mental health in a population-based survey of New Zealand adolescents and adults, *American Journal of Clinical Nutrition* 86 (2007): 1278–1285.

M. Lucas, G. Asselin, C. Mérette et al., Ethyl-eicosapentaenoic acid for the treatment of psychological distress and depressive symptoms in middle-aged women: A double-blind, placebo-controlled, randomized clinical trial, *American Journal of Clinical Nutrition* 89 (2009): 641–651; M. Maes, A. Christophe, E. Bosmans et al., In humans, serum polyunsaturated fatty acid levels predict the response of proinflammatory cytokines to psychologic stress, *Biological Psychiatry* 47 (2000): 910–920; E. Albanese, A. D. Dangour, R. Uauy et al., Dietary fish and meat intake and dementia in Latin America, China, and India, *American Journal of Clinical Nutrition* 90 (2009): 392–400.

13. M. P. Freeman, J. R. Hibbeln, K. L. Wisner et al., Omega-3 fatty acids: Evidence basis for treatment and future research in psychiatry, *Journal of Clinical Psychiatry* 67 (2006): 1954–1967.

14. M. Lafourcade, T. Larrieu, S. Mato et al., Nutritional omega-3 deficiency abolishes endocannabinoid-mediated neuronal functions, *Nature Neuroscience* 14 (2011): 345–350.

15. W. E. Lands, *Fish, Omega-3 and Human Health*, 2d ed. (AOCS Books, 2005).

16. M. D. Lewis, J. R. Hibbeln, J. E. Johnson et al., Suicide deaths of active-duty U.S. military and omega-3 fatty-acid status: A case-control comparison, *Journal of Clinical Psychiatry* 72 (2011): 1585–1590.

17. K. Kendall-Tackett, Personal communication, May 2011; K. Kendall-Tackett, ed., *The Psychoneuroimmunology of Chronic Disease: Exploring the Links Between Inflammation, Stress, and Illness* (American Psychological Association, 2009).

18. J. K. Kiecolt-Glaser, M. A. Belury, R. Andridge et al., Omega-3 supplementation lowers inflammation and anxiety in medical students: A randomized controlled trial, *Brain, Behavior, and Immunity* 25 (2011): 1725–1734.

19. These studies found omega-3 benefits for brain health. M. F. Muldoon, C. M. Ryan, L. Sheu et al., Serum phospholipid docosahexaenonic acid is associated with cognitive functioning during middle adulthood, *Journal of Nutrition* 140 (2010): 848–853; K. Yurko-Mauro, D. McCarthy, D. Rom et al., Beneficial effects of docosahexaenoic acid on cognition in age-related cognitive decline, *Alzheimer's and Dementia* 6 (2010): 456–464; K. Yurko-Mauro et al., Cognitive and cardiovascular benefits of docosahexaenoic acid in aging and cognitive decline, *Current Alzheimer Research* 7 (2010): 190–196.

   This study found that supplementation with DHA did not slow the rate of cognitive and functional decline in Alzheimer's patients. J. F. Quinn, R. Raman, R. G. Thomas et al., Docosahexaenolic acid supplementation and cognitive decline in Alzheimer disease: A randomized trial, *JAMA* 304 (2010): 1903–1911.

20. B. M. van Gelder, M. Tijhuis, S. Kalmijn et al., Fish consumption, n-3 fatty acids, and subsequent 5-year cognitive decline in elderly men: The Zutphen elderly study, *American Journal of Clinical Nutrition* 85 (2007): 1142–1147.

21. S. Jazayeri, M. Tehrani-Doost, S. A. Keshavarz et al., Comparison of therapeutic effects of omega-3 fatty acid eicosapentaenoic acid and fluoxetine, separately and in combination, in major depressive disorder, *Australian and New Zealand Journal of Psychiatry* 42 (2008): 192–198.

22. G. P. Amminger, M. R. Schäfer, K. Papageorgiou et al., Long-chain omega-3 fatty acids for indicated prevention of psychiatric disorders, *Archives of General Psychiatry* 67 (2010): 146–154.

23. J. A. Blumenthal, M. A. Babyak, P. M. Doraiswamy et al., Exercise and pharmacotherapy in the treatment of major depressive disorder, *Psychosomatic Medicine* 69 (2007): 587–596; M. Hamer and A. Steptoe,

Association between physical fitness, parasympathetic control, and proinflammatory responses to mental stress, *Psychosomatic Medicine* 69 (2007): 660–666.

Chapter 5 How Omega-3s Help Childhood Ds

1. A. J. Richardson and P. Montgomery, The Oxford-Durham Study: A randomized, controlled trial of dietary supplementation with fatty acids in children with developmental coordination disorder, *Pediatrics* 115 (2005): 1360–1366. (The handwriting samples are from the supplemental data file, not the main article.)
2. R. K. McNamara, J. Able, R. Jandacek et al., Docosahexaenoic acid supplementation increases prefrontal cortex activation during sustained attention in healthy boys: A placebo-controlled, dose-ranging, functional magnetic resonance imaging study, *American Journal of Clinical Nutrition* 91 (2010): 1060–1067.
3. S. M. Madden, C. F. Garrioch, and B. J. Holub, Direct diet quantification indicates low intakes of (n-3) fatty acids in children 4 to 8 years old, *Journal of Nutrition* 139 (2009): 528–532.
4. G. Meiri, Y. Bichovsky, and R. H. Belmaker, Omega-3 fatty acid treatment in autism, *Journal of Child and Adolescent Psychopharmacology* 19 (2009): 449–451.
5. P. A. Gustafsson, U. Birberg-Thornberg, K. Duchén et al., EPA supplementation improves teacher-rated behaviour and oppositional symptoms in children with ADHD, *Acta Paediatrica* 99 (2010): 1540–1549.
6. M. H. Bloch and A. Qawasmi, Omega-3 fatty acid supplementation for the treatment of children with attention-deficit/hyperactivity disorder symptomatology: Systematic review and meta-analysis, *Journal of the American Academy of Child and Adolescent Psychiatry* 50 (2011): 991–1000. See also N. Vaisman, N. Kaysar, Y. Zaruk-Adasha et al., Correlation between changes in blood fatty acid composition and visual sustained attention performance in children with inattention: Effect of dietary n-3 fatty acids containing phospholipids, *American Journal of Clinical Nutrition* 87 (2008): 1170–1180; N. Sinn and J. Bryan, Effect of supplementation with polyunsaturated fatty acid and micronutrients on learning and behavior problems associated with child ADHD, *Journal of Developmental and Behavioral Pediatrics* 28 (2007): 82–91.

Not all studies showed benefits of omega-3 supplements on ADHD symptoms. R. Raz and L. Gabis, Essential fatty acids and attention-deficit-hyperactivity disorder: A systematic review, *Developmental Medicine and Child Neurology* 51 (2009): 580–592.

7. Blaylock Wellness Report, 2 (April 2005): 5; L. J. Stevens, S. S. Zentall, M. L. Abate et al., Omega-3 fatty acids in boys with behavior, learning, and health problems, *Physiology and Behavior* 59 (1996): 915–920.

8. T. Hamazaki, S. Sawazaki, M. Itomura et al., The effect of docosahexaenoic acid on aggression in young adults: A placebo-controlled double-blind study, *Journal of Clinical Investigation* 97 (1996): 1129–1133.

9. L. Lindmark and P. Clough, A five-month open study with long-chain polyunsaturated fatty acids in dyslexia, *Journal of Medicinal Food* 10 (2007): 662–666.

Chapter 6 Enjoy the Omega-3 Effect during Pregnancy and Your Child's Infancy

1. S. E. Carlson, Docosahexaenoic acid supplementation in pregnancy and lactation, *American Journal of Clinical Nutrition* 89 (2009): S678–S684; J. Farquharson, Infant cerebral cortex and dietary fatty acids, *European Journal of Clinical Nutrition* 48 (1994): S24–S25; M. Makrides and R. A. Gibson, Long-chain polyunsaturated fatty acid requirements during pregnancy and lactation, *American Journal of Clinical Nutrition* 71 (2008): 3075–3115; J. C. Kent, L. R. Mitoulas, M. D. Cregan et al., Volume and frequency of breastfeedings and fat content of breast milk throughout the day, *Pediatrics* 117 (2006): e387–e395; R. G. Jensen, C. J. Lammi-Keefe, R. A. Henderson et al. Effect of dietary intake of n-6 and n-3 fatty acids on the fatty acid composition of human milk in North America, *Journal of Pediatrics* 120 (1992): 587–592; W. M. Ratnayake and Z. Y. Chen, Trans, n-3, and n-6 fatty acids in Canadian human milk, *Lipids* 31 (1996): S279–S282; L. J. Horwood and D. M. Fergusson, Breastfeeding and later cognitive and academic outcomes, *Pediatrics* 101 (1998): e9.

Studies measuring blood fats of women during pregnancy found that the levels of omega-3 fats fell during pregnancy, and the deficiency persisted until at least six weeks after delivery. The DHA level fell the most, but ALA and EPA levels also fell. The article concluded that dietary supplementation might be indicated. R. T. Holman, S. B.

Johnson, and P. L. Ogburn, Deficiency of essential fatty acids and membrane fluidity during pregnancy and lactation, *Proceedings of the National Academy of Sciences* 88 (1991): 4835–4839.

2. M. A. Williams, R. W. Zingheim, I. B. King et al., Omega-3 fatty acids in maternal erythrocytes and risk of preeclampsia, *Epidemiology* 6 (1995): 232–237; C. Qiu, S. E. Sanchez, G. Larrabure et al., Erythrocyte omega-3 and omega-6 polyunsaturated fatty acids and preeclampsia risk in Peruvian women, *Archives of Gynecology and Obstetrics* 274 (2006): 97–103.

3. J. S. Radesky, E. Oken, S. L. Rifas-Shiman et al., Diet during early pregnancy and development of gestational diabetes, *Paediatric and Perinatal Epidemiology* 22 (2008): 47–59.

4. C. M Smuts, M. Huang, D. Mundy et al., A randomized trial of DHA supplementation during the third trimester of pregnancy, *Obstetrics and Gynecology* 101 (2003): 469–479.

5. B. M. Leung and B. J. Kaplan, Perinatal depression: Prevalence, risks, and the nutrition link, *Journal of the American Dietetic Association* 109 (2009): 1566–1575; J. R. Hibbeln, Seafood consumption, the DHA content of mothers' milk and prevalence rates of postpartum depression, *Journal of Affective Disorders* 69 (2002): 15–29; K. Kendall-Tackett, Personal communication, May 2011; K. Kendall-Tackett, A new paradigm for depression in new mothers: The central role of inflammation and how breastfeeding and anti-inflammatory treatments protect maternal mental health, *International Breastfeeding Journal* 2 (2007): 1–14.

This study did not substantiate a clear link between postpartum depression and fish and n-3 fatty acid intake. Y. Miyake, S. Sasaki, T. Yokoyama et al., Risk of postpartum depression in relation to dietary fish and fat intake in Japan: The Osaka Maternal and Child Health Study, *Psychological Medicine* 36 (2006): 1727–1735.

In this study, the authors concluded there is little evidence to support an association between dietary omega-3 intake and postpartum depression. Yet, the data show that more mothers needed medication in the lowest omega-3 intake group. M. Strøm, E. L. Mortensen, T. I. Halldorsson et al., Fish and long-chain n-3 polyunsaturated fatty acid intakes during pregnancy and risk of postpartum depression: A prospective study based on a large national birth cohort, *American Journal of Clinical Nutrition* 90 (2009): 149–155.

6. J. Colombo, K. N. Kannass, D. J. Shaddy et al., Maternal DHA and the development of attention in infancy and toddlerhood, *Child Development* 75 (2004): 1254–1267.

7. B. Alm, N. Aberg, L. Erdes et al., Early introduction of fish decreases the risk of eczema in infants, *Archives of Disease in Childhood* 94 (2009): 11–15; C. Furuhjelm, K. Warstedt, J. Larsson et al., Fish oil supplementation in pregnancy and lactation may decrease the risk of infant allergy, *Acta Paediatrica* 98 (2009): 1461–1467.

    In a sixteen-year follow-up of five hundred children whose mothers took fish oil supplements during pregnancy, the rate of asthma was reduced by 87 percent. S. F. Olsen, M. L. Ûsterdal, J. D. Salvig et al., Fish oil intake compared with olive oil intake in late pregnancy and asthma in the offspring, *American Journal of Clinical Nutrition* 88 (2008): 167–175.

8. S. R. Cheruku, H. E. Montgomery-Downs, S. L. Farkas et al., Higher maternal plasma DHA during pregnancy is associated with more mature neonatal sleep-states patterning, *American Journal of Clinical Nutrition* 76 (2002): 608–613.

9. I. B. Helland, L. Smith, and K. Saarem et al., Maternal supplementation with very-long-chain n-3 fatty acids during pregnancy and lactation augments children's IQ at 4 years of age, *Pediatrics* 111 (2003): e39–e44; J. R. Hibbeln, J. M. Davis, C. Steer et al., Maternal seafood consumption in pregnancy and neurodevelopmental outcomes in childhood (ALSPAC study), *Lancet* 369 (2007): 578–585; J. Colombo, K. N. Kannass, D. J. Shaddy et al., Maternal DHA and the development of attention in infancy and toddlerhood, *Child Development* 75 (2004): 1254–1267; J. W. Anderson, B. M. Johnstone, and D. T. Remley, Breast-feeding and cognitive development: A meta-analysis, *American Journal of Clinical Nutrition* 70 (1999): 525–535.

10. S. F. Olsen, H. S. Hansen, T. I. Sørensen et al., Intake of marine fat, rich in (n-3) polyunsaturated fatty acids, may increase birthweight by prolonging gestation, *Lancet* 2 (1986): 367–369; S. F. Olsen, J. D. Sorensen, N. J. Secher et al., Randomised controlled trial of effect of fish oil supplementation on pregnancy duration, *Lancet* 339 (1992): 1003–1007.

11. M. Maes, A. H. Lin, W. Ombelet et al., Immune activation in the early puerperium is related to postpartum anxiety and depressive symptoms, *Psychoneuroendocrinology* (2000): 25:121–137.

12. I. B. Helland, L. Smith, and K. Saarem et al., Maternal supplementation with very-long-chain n-3 fatty acids during pregnancy and lactation augments children's IQ at 4 years of age, *Pediatrics* 111 (2003): e39–e44.

13. S. R. Cheruku, H. E. Montgomery-Downs, S. L. Farkas et al., Higher maternal plasma DHA during pregnancy is associated with more mature neonatal sleep-states patterning, *American Journal of Clinical Nutrition* 76 (2002): 608–613.

14. M. S. Kramer, F. Aboud, E. Mironova et al., Breastfeeding and child cognitive development: New evidence from a large randomised trial, *Archives of General Psychology* 65 (2008): 578–584.

15. C. L. Jensen, Effects of n-3 fatty acids during pregnancy and lactation, *American Journal of Clinical Nutrition* 83 (2006): S1452–S1457; B. Koletzko, I. Thiel, and P. O. Abiodun, The fatty acid content of human milk in Europe and Africa, *Journal of Pediatrics* 120 (1992): 562–570.

16. R. Yuhas, K. Pramuk, and E. L. Lien, Human milk fatty acid composition from nine countries varies most in DHA, *Lipids* 41 (2006): 851–858.

17. R. W. Byard, M. Makrides, M. Need et al., Sudden infant death syndrome: Effect of breast and formula feeding on frontal cortex and brainstem lipid composition, *Journal of Paediatrics and Child Health* 31 (1995): 14–16; M. Makrides, M. A. Neumann, R. W. Byard et al., Fatty acid composition of brain, retina, and erythrocytes in breast and formula-fed infants, *American Journal of Clinical Nutrition* 60 (1994): 189–194; E. C. Jamieson, J. Farquharson, R. W. Logan et al., Infant cerebellar gray and white matter fatty acids in relation to age and diet, *Lipids* 34 (1999): 1065–1071; J. Farquharson, F. Cockburn, W. A. Patrick et al., Infant cerebral cortex phospholipid fatty-acid composition and diet, *Lancet* 340 (1992): 810–813; J. Farquharson, E. C. Jamieson, K. A. Abbasi et al., Effect of diet on the fatty acid composition of the major phospholipids of infant cerebral cortex, Archives of Disease in Childhood 72 (1995): 198–203.

18. J. A. Attaman, T. L. Toth, J. Furtado et al., Dietary fat and semen quality among men attending a fertility clinic, *Human Reproduction* 27 (2012): 1466–1474.

19. M. Roqueta-Rivera, T. L. Abbott, M. Sivaguru et al., Deficiency in the omega-3 fatty acid pathway results in failure of acrosome biogenesis in mice, *Biology of Reproduction* 85 (2011): 721–732.

20. C. L. Jensen, Effects of n-3 fatty acids during pregnancy and lactation, *American Journal of Clinical Nutrition* 83 (2006): S1452–S1457; E. L. Lien, Toxicology and safety of DHA, *Prostaglandins, Leukotrienes and Essential Fatty Acids* 81 (2009): 125–132; E. L. Lien, Personal communication, September 2011; J. A. Greenberg, S. J. Bell, and W. Van Ausdal, Omega-3 fatty acid supplementation during pregnancy, *Obstetrics and Gynecology* 1 (2008): 162–169.

21. E. L. Lien, Toxicology and safety of DHA, *Prostaglandins, Leukotrienes and Essential Fatty Acids* 81 (2009): 125–132; E. L. Lien, Personal communication, September 2011.

Chapter 7 How Omega-3s Help *-itis* Illnesses

1. J. C. Maroon and J. W. Bost, Omega-3 fatty acids (fish oil) as an anti-inflammatory: An alternative to nonsteroidal anti-inflammatory drugs for discogenic pain, *Surgical Neurology* 65 (2006): 326–331.

2. C. T. Damsgaard, L. Lauritzen, T. M. Kjær et al., Fish oil supplementation modulates immune function in healthy infants, *Journal of Nutrition* 137 (2007): 1031–1036.

3. This study concluded that supplementation with n-3 fatty acids may be helpful in the case of irritable bowel syndrome. T. Solakivi, K. Kaukinen, T. Kunnas et al., Serum fatty acid profile in subjects with irritable bowel syndrome, *Scandinavian Journal of Gastroenterology* 46 (2011): 299–303.

This study showed that patients supplemented with 2.7 grams of omega-3s showed a reduced rate of relapse in Crohn's disease. A. Belluzzi, C. Brignola, M. Campieri et al., Effect of an enteric-coated fish-oil preparation on relapses in Crohn's disease, *New England Journal of Medicine* 334 (1996): 1557–1560.

This study concluded that omega-3 supplements did not prevent relapse in Crohn's disease. B. G. Feagan, W. J. Sandborn, U. Mittmann et al., Omega-3 fatty acids for the maintenance of remission in Crohn disease: The EPIC randomized controlled trials, *JAMA* 299 (2008): 1690–1697.

4. R. Schubert, R. Kitz, C. Beermann et al., Effect of n-3 polyunsaturated fatty acids in asthma after low-dose allergen challenge, *International Archives of Allergy and Immunology* 148 (2009): 321–329.

5. J. M. Norris, X. Yin, M. M. Lamb et al., Omega-3 polyunsaturated fatty acid intake and islet autoimmunity in children at increased risk for type 1 diabetes, *JAMA* 298 (2007): 1420–1428. Regarding type 2

diabetes in adults, see A. Stirban, S. Nandrean, C. Götting et al., Effects of n-3 fatty acids on macro- and microvascular function in subjects with type 2 diabetes mellitus, *American Journal of Clinical Nutrition* 91 (2010): 808–813; R. J. Woodman, T. A. Mori, V. Burke et al., Docosahexaenoic acid but not eicosapentaenoic acid increases LDL particle size in treated hypertensive type 2 diabetic patients, *Diabetes Care* 26 (2003): 253 (letter).

6. A. O. Akinkuolie, J. S. Ngwa, J. B. Meigs et al., Omega-3 polyunsaturated fatty acid and insulin sensitivity: A meta-analysis of randomized controlled trials, *Clinical Nutrition* 30 (2011): 702–707.

7. E. K. Kaye, n-3 fatty acid intake and periodontal disease, *Journal of the American Dietetic Association* 110 (2010): 1650–1652. See also A. Z. Naqvi, C. Buettner, R. S. Phillips et al., n-3 fatty acids and periodontitis in U.S. adults, *Journal of the American Dietetic Association* 110 (2010): 1669–1675.

8. H. Hasturk, A. Kantarci, E. Goguet-Surmenian et al., Resolvin E1 regulates inflammation at the cellular and tissue level and restores tissue homeostasis in vivo, *Journal of Immunology* 179 (2007): 7021–7029; L. Kesavalu, B. Vasudevan, B. Raghu et al., Omega-3 fatty acid effect on alveolar bone loss in rats, *Journal of Dental Research* 85 (2006): 648–652.

9. C. Koch, S. Dölle, M. Metzger et al., Docosahexaenoic acid (DHA) supplementation in atopic eczema: A randomized, double-blind, controlled trial, *British Journal of Dermatology* 158 (2008): 786–792; B. Alm, N. Aberg, L. Erdes et al., Early introduction of fish decreases the risk of eczema in infants, *Archives of Disease in Childhood* 94 (2009): 11–15; C. Furuhjelm, K. Warstedt, J. Larsson et al., Fish oil supplementation in pregnancy and lactation may decrease the risk of infant allergy, *Acta Paediatrica* 98 (2009): 1461–1467.

Chapter 8 How Omega-3s Help You Lose Weight

1. T. L. Blasbalg, J. R. Hibbeln, C. E. Ramsden et al., Changes in consumption of omega-3 and omega-6 fatty acids in the United States during the twentieth century, *American Journal of Clinical Nutrition* 93 (2011): 950–962.

2. M. Itoh, T. Suganami, N. Satoh et al., Increased adiponectin secretion by highly purified eicosapentaenoic acid in rodent models of obesity and human obese subjects, *Arteriosclerosis, Thrombosis, and Vascular*

Biology 9 (2007): 1918–1925; M. Micallef, I. Munro, M. Phang et al., Plasma n-3 polyunsaturated fatty acids are negatively associated with obesity, *British Journal of Nutrition* 102 (2009): 1370–1374; J. D. Buckley and P. R. Howe, Anti-obesity effects of long-chain omega-3 polyunsaturated fatty acids, *Obesity Reviews* 10 (2009): 648–659; A. González-Périz, R. Horrillo, N. Ferré et al., Obesity-induced insulin resistance and hepatic steatosis are alleviated by omega-3 fatty acids: A role for resolvins and protectins, *FASEB Journal* 23 (2009): 1946–1957.

   A study showed that obese Inuits who traditionally eat a lot of omega-3 EPA/DHA tend to have a lower incidence of obesity-causing metabolic syndrome than non-Inuit obese controls. This finding led researchers to conclude that omega-3 EPA/DHA may somewhat lessen the severity of metabolic syndrome in already obese persons. Z. Makhoul, A. R. Kristal, R. Gulati et al., Associations of obesity with triglycerides and C-reactive protein are attenuated in adults with high red blood cell eicosapentaenoic and docosahexaenoic acids, *European Journal of Clinical Nutrition* 65 (2011): 808–817.

   Another study found that omega-3 EPA/DHA has a positive influence on levels of HDL, the "good cholesterol." E. E. Dewailly, C. Blanchet, S. Gingras et al., Relations between n-3 fatty acid status and cardiovascular disease risk factors among Quebecers, *American Journal of Clinical Nutrition* 74 (2001): 603–611.

3. Y. A. Carpentier, L. Portois, and W. J. Malaisse, n-3 fatty acids and the metabolic syndrome, *American Journal of Clinical Nutrition* 83 (2006): S1499–S1504.

4. A. M. Hill, Combining fish-oil supplements with regular aerobic exercise improves body composition and cardiovascular disease risk factors, *American Journal of Clinical Nutrition* 85 (2007): 1267–1274.

5. T. Burrows, C. E. Collins, and M. L. Garg, Omega-3 index, obesity and insulin resistance in children, *International Journal of Pediatric Obesity* 6 (2011): e532–e539; S. C. Savva, C. Chadjigeorgiou, C. Hatzis et al., Association of adipose tissue arachidonic acid content with BMI and overweight status in children from Cyprus and Crete, *British Journal of Nutrition* 91 (2004): 643–649.

6. D. Parra, A. Ramel, N. Bandarra et al., A diet rich in long chain omega-3 fatty acids modulates satiety in overweight and obese volunteers during weight loss, *Appetite* 51 (2008): 676–680.

7 D. Parra, A. Ramel, N. Bandarra et al., A diet rich in long chain omega-3 fatty acids modulates satiety in overweight and obese volunteers during weight loss, *Appetite* 51 (2008): 676–680.

8. L. F. DeFina, L. G. Marcoux, S. M. Devers et al., Effects of omega-3 supplementation in combination with diet and exercise on weight loss and body composition, *American Journal of Clinical Nutrition* 93 (2011): 455–462.

Chapter 9 How Omega-3s Help Keep You Young

1. G. Bartzokis, Personal communication, June 2011; G. Bartzokis, Neuroglialpharmacology: White matter and psychiatric treatments, *Frontiers in Bioscience* 17 (2011): 2695–2733.

2. S. H. Lee, M. J. Shin, J. S. Kim et al., Blood eicosapentaenoic acid and docosahexaenoic acid as predictors of all-cause mortality in patients with acute myocardial infarction, *Circulation Journal* 73 (2009): 2250–2257; J. H. O'Keefe, H. Abuissa, A. Sastre et al., Effects of omega-3 fatty acids on resting heart rate, heart rate recovery after exercise, and heart rate variability in men with healed myocardial infarctions and depressed ejection fractions, *American Journal of Cardiology* 97 (2008): 1127–1130.

   A forty-year study of 1,373 men born between 1900 and 1920 found that the longer the men had been eating at least 250 mg per day of fish oil, the more their risk of cardiovascular disease decreased. M. T. Streppel, M. C. Ockél, H. C. Boshuizen et al., Long-term fish consumption and n-3 fatty acid intake in relation to (sudden) coronary heart disease death: The Zutphen study, *European Heart Journal* 29 (2008): 2024–2030.

3. H. Iso, K. M. Rexrode, M. J. Stampfer et al., Intake of fish and omega-3 fatty acids and risk of stroke in women, *JAMA* 285 (2001): 304–312; M. Lalancette-Hébert, C. Julien, P. Cordeau et al., Accumulation of dietary docosahexaenoic acid in the brain attenuates acute immune response and development of postischemic neuronal damage, *Stroke* 42 (2011): 2903–2909; L. Belayev, V. L. Marcheselli, L. Khoutorova et al., Docosahexaenoic acid complexed to albumin elicits high-grade ischemic neuroprotection, *Stroke* 36 (2005): 118–123.

   Men who ate an average of an ounce of fish per day suffered half the number of strokes compared to those who ate less. K. He, Y. Song, M. L. Daviglus et al., Fish consumption and incidence of stroke: A meta-analysis of cohort studies, *Stroke* 35 (2001): 1538–1542.

4. R. Uauy and A. D. Dangour, Nutrition in brain development and aging: Role of essential fatty acids, *Nutrition Reviews* 64 (2006): S24–S33.

5. E. Kesse-Guyot, S. Péneau, M. Ferry et al., Thirteen-year prospective study between fish consumption, long-chain n-3 fatty acid intakes and cognitive function, *Journal of Nutrition Health Aging* 15 (2011): 115–120; S. Kalmijn, E. J. Feskens, L J. Launer et al., Polyunsaturated fatty acids, antioxidants, and cognitive function in very old men, *American Journal of Epidemiology* 145 (1997): 33–41; G. Bartzokis, Neuroglialpharmacology: White matter and psychiatric treatments, *Frontiers in Bioscience* 17 (2011): 2695–2733.

6. M. Rondanelli, A. Giacosa, A. Opizzi et al., Long-chain omega-3 polyunsaturated fatty acids supplementation in the treatment of elderly depression: Effects on depressive symptoms, on phospholipids fatty acids profile and on health-related quality of life, *Journal of Nutrition Health Aging* 15 (2011): 37–44; Y. Tajalizadekhoob, F. Sharifi, H. Fakhrzadeh et al., The effect of low-dose omega-3 fatty acids on the treatment of mild to moderate depression in the elderly: A double-blind, randomized, placebo-controlled study, *European Archives of Psychiatry and Clinical Neuroscience* 261 (2011): 539–549.

7. E. J. Johnson, H. Y. Chung, S. M. Caldarella et al., The influence of supplemental lutein and docosahexaenoic acid on serum, lipoproteins, and macular pigmentation, *American Journal of Clinical Nutrition* 87 (2008): 1521–1529; J. P. Sangiovanni, E. Agrón, A. D. Meleth et al., Omega-3 long-chain polyunsaturated fatty acid intake and 12–year incidence of neovascular age-related macular degeneration and central geographic atrophy: AREDS report 30, a prospective cohort study from the age-related eye disease study, *American Journal of Clinical Nutrition* 90 (2009): 1601–1607.

8. E. K. Kaye, n-3 fatty acid intake and periodontal disease, *Journal of the American Dietetic Association* 110 (2010): 1650–1652; A. Z. Nacvi, C. Buettner, R. S. Phillips et al., n-3 fatty acids and periodontitis in U.S. adults, *Journal of the American Dietetic Association* 110 (2010): 1669–1675; H. Hasturk, A. Kantarci, E. Goguet-Surmenian et al., Resolvin E1 regulates inflammation at the cellular and tissue level and restores tissue homeostasis in vivo, *Journal of Immunology* 179 (2007): 7021–7029; L. Kesavalu, B. Vasudevan, B. Raghu et al., Omega-3 fatty acid effect on alveolar bone loss in rats, *Journal of Dental Research* 85 (2006): 648–652.

9. B. Gopinath, V. M. Flood, E. Rochtchina et al., Consumption of omega-3 fatty acids and fish and risk of age-related hearing loss, *American Journal of Clinical Nutrition* 92 (2010): 416–421.

10. M. Högström, P. Nordström, and A. Nordström, n-3 fatty acids are positively associated with peak bone mineral density and bone accrual in healthy men: The NO$_2$ study, *American Journal of Clinical Nutrition* 85 (2007): 803–807.

11. M. Lindberg, I. Saltvedt, O. Sletvold et al., Long-chain n-3 fatty acids and mortality in elderly patients, *American Journal of Clinical Nutrition* 88 (2008): 722–729.

12. M. Fossel, G. Blackburn, and D. Woynarowski, *The Immortality Edge* (Wiley, 2010).

13. R. Farzaneh-Far, J. Lin, E. S. Epel et al., Association of marine omega-3 fatty acid levels with telomeric aging in patients with coronary heart disease, *JAMA* 303 (2010): 250–257.

14. D. Ornish, J. Lin, J. Daubenmier et al., Increased telomerase activity and comprehensive lifestyle changes, *Lancet Oncology* 9 (2008): 1048–1057.

Chapter 10 How Omega-3s Help You Heal

1. These studies show how omega-3s support healing in a variety of ways. R. E. Ward, W. Huang, O. E. Curran et al., Docosahexaenoic acid prevents white matter damage after spinal cord injury, *Journal of Neurotrauma* 27 (2010): 1769–1780; G. Mariscalco, S. Sarzi Braga, M. Banach et al., Preoperative n-3 polyunsatured fatty acids are associated with a decrease in the incidence of early atrial fibrillation following cardiac surgery, *Angiology* 61 (2010): 643–650; L. Calò, L. Bianconi, F. Colivicchi et al., n-3 fatty acids for the prevention of atrial fibrillation after coronary artery bypass surgery, *Journal of the American College of Cardiology* 45 (2005): 1723–1728; G. J. Dehmer, J. J. Popma, E. K. van den Berg et al., Reduction in the rate of early restenosis after coronary angioplasty by a diet supplemented with n-3 fatty acids, *New England Journal of Medicine* 319 (1988): 733–740; X. Wang, W. Li, N. L. et al., Omega-3 fatty acid-supplemented parental nutrition decreases hyperinflammatory response and attenuates systemic disease sequelae in severe pancreatitis: A randomized and controlled study. *Journal of Parenteral and Enteral Nutrition* 32 (2008): 236–241; R. Saynor, D. Verel, and T. Gillott, The long-term effects of dietary

supplementation of fish oil concentrate on serum lipids, bleeding time, platelets, and angina, *Atherosclerosis* 50 (1984): 3–10.

2. S. R. Erdely, The government's big fish story, *Men's Health,* June 21, 2007. Available at www.menshealth.com.

3. Nutritional Armor for the Warfighter. Conference at the National Institutes of Health, October 13, 2009.

4. Nutritional Armor for the Warfighter: Can Omega-3 Fatty Acids Enhance Resilience, Wellness, and Military Performance? Conference at the National Institutes of Health, October 13, 2009. A videocast is available at http://videocast.nih.gov/summary.asp?live=8107.

5. J. T. Brenna, Personal communication, December 2011; J. P. Infante, R. C. Kirwan, and J. T. Brenna, High levels of docosahexaenoic acid (22:6n-3)-containing phospholipids in high-frequency contraction muscles of hummingbirds and rattlesnakes, *Comparative Biochemistry and Physiology Part B* 130 (2001): 291–298.

Part III Selecting Fish Oil Supplements and Enjoying Safe Seafood

1. Chinese Nutrition Society Meeting, May 2010.

Chapter 11 Getting the Most Omega-3 Effect out of Omega-3 Supplements

1. These authors cite the scientific basis for the recommendation of 500 mg per day of omega-3 EPA/DHA. An average daily dose of 566 mg reduced the risk of coronary heart disease by 37 percent. W. S. Harris, P. M. Kris-Etherton, and K. A. Harris, Intakes of long-chain omega-3 fatty acid associated with reduced risk for death from coronary heart disease in healthy adults, *Current Atherosclerosis Reports* 10 (2008): 503–509.

The International Society for the Study of Fatty Acids and Lipids (ISSFAL) recommends a minimum of 500 mg per day. The National Institutes of Health (1999) recommends that EPA/DHA intake should equal 650 mg per day, with DHA at least 220 mg per day and EPA at least 220 mg per day.

2. J. R. Hibbeln, L. Nieminen, T. L. Blasbalg et al., Healthy intakes of n-3 and n-6 fatty acids: Estimations considering worldwide diversity, *American Journal of Clinical Nutrition* 83 (2006): S1483–S1493.

3. "Patients with coronary heart disease should be encouraged to increase their consumption of EPA and DHA to approximately 1 gram

[1000 mg] per day, which is the dose used in the GISSI-Prevention Study." P. M. Kris-Etherton, W. S. Harris, and L. J. Appel, for the Nutrition Committee of the American Heart Association, AHA scientific statement: Fish consumption, fish oil, omega-3 fatty acids, and cardiovascular disease, *Arteriosclerosis, Thrombosis, and Vascular Biology* 23 (2003): e20–e30.

R. Marchioli, F. Barzi, E. Bomba et al., Dietary supplementation with n-3 polyunsaturated fatty acids and vitamin E after myocardial infarction: Results of the GISSI-Prevenzione trial, *Lancet* 354 (Aug. 7, 1999): 447–455; R. Marchioli, F. Barzi, E. Bomba et al., Early protection against sudden death by n-3 polyunsaturated fatty acids after myocardial infarction: Time-course analysis of the results of the GISSI-Prevenzione study, *Circulation* 105 (2002): 1897–1903.

4. "Patients needing triglyceride lowering [should take] 2000–4000 mg (2–4 grams) of EPA+DHA per day, provided as capsules under a physician's care." P. M. Kris-Etherton, W. S. Harris, and L. J. Appel, for the Nutrition Committee of the American Heart Association, AHA scientific statement: Fish consumption, fish oil, omega-3 fatty acids, and cardiovascular disease, *Arteriosclerosis, Thrombosis, and Vascular Biology* 23 (2003): e20–e30.

5. Food and Agriculture Organization of the United Nations, Fat and fatty acid intake and inflammatory and immune response: Rheumatoid arthritis, in *Fats and Fatty Acids in Human Nutrition: Report of an Expert Consultation* (2008), 95; P. C. Calder, Polyunsaturated fatty acids and inflammation: Therapeutic potential in rheumatoid arthritis, *Current Rheumatology Reviews* 5 (2009): 214–225.

6. Dr. William Harris, Personal communication, December 2010.

7. L. M. Arterburn, E. B. Hall, and H. Oken, Distribution, interconversion, and dose response of n-3 fatty acids in humans, *American Journal of Clinical Nutrition* 83 (2006): S1467–S1476.

8. G. C. Burdge and S. A. Wootton, Conversion of alpha-linolenic acid to eicosapentaenoic, docosapentaenoic, and docosahexaenoic acids in young women, *British Journal of Nutrition* 88 (2002): 411–420; A. P. Kitson, C. K. Stroud, and K. D. Stark, Elevated production of docosahexaenoic acid in females: Potential molecular mechanisms, *Lipids* 45 (2010): 209–224.

9. This article reviews the current scientific studies on krill oil. J. Ramirez, Krill oil optimizes multimodal arthritis control, *Life Extension Magazine*, November 2011, www.lef.org.

10. A. P. Simopoulos and N. Salem Jr., n-3 fatty acids in eggs from range-fed Greek chickens, *New England Journal of Medicine* 321 (1989): 1412 (letter); A. P. Simopoulos and N. Salem Jr., Egg yolk as a source of long-chain polyunsaturated fatty acids in infant feeding, *American Journal of Clinical Nutrition* 55 (1992): 411–414.

11. Dr. William Harris, Personal communication, August 2011.

12. An animal study, in which omega-3 decreased by 17 percent (and omega-6 increased) in alcohol-exposed animals, concluded that loss in nervous system function may underlie some of the neuropathy associated with alcoholism. R. J. Pawlosky and N. Salem Jr., Ethanol exposure causes a decrease in docosahexaenoic acid and an increase in docosapentaenoic acid in feline brains and retinas, *American Journal of Clinical Nutrition* 61 (1995): 1284–1289. See also D. F. Horrobin, Essential fatty acids, prostaglandins, and alcoholism: An overview, *Alcoholism: Clinical and Experimental Research* 11 (1987): 2–9.

13. T. Norat, S. Bingham, P. Ferrari et al., Meat, fish, and colorectal cancer risk: The European prospective investigation into cancer and nutrition, *Journal of the National Cancer Institute* 97 (2005): 906–916.

14. E. Theodoratou, G. McNeill, R. Cetnarskyj et al., Dietary fatty acids and colorectal cancer: A case-control study, *American Journal of Epidemiology* 166 (2007): 181–195.

Other studies found that omega-3s may be of use in preventing colon cancer and bowel disease. C. E. Roynette, P. C. Calder, Y. M. Dupertuis et al., n-3 polyunsaturated fatty acids and colon cancer prevention, *Clinical Nutrition* 23 (2004): 139–151; Y. C. Huang, J. M. Jessup, R. A. Forse et al., n-3 fatty acids decrease colonic epithelial cell proliferation in high-risk bowel mucosa, *Lipids* 31 (1996): S313–S317.

15. M. N. Phillips, J. Chavarro, M. Stampfer et al., A prospective study of fish, n-3 fatty acid intake, and colorectal cancer risk in men, in *Proceedings of the Fifth AACR International Conference on Frontiers in Cancer Prevention Research,* April 2006 (abstract B165).

16. N. J. West, S. K. Clark, R. K. Phillips et al., Eicosapentaenoic acid reduces rectal polyp number and size in familial adenomatous polyposis, *GUT* 59 (2010): 918–925.

17. M. Hedelin, E. T. Chang, F. Wiklund et al., Association of frequent consumption of fatty fish with prostate cancer risk is modified by COX-2 polymorphism, *International Journal of Cancer* 120 (2007): 398–405.

Another Swedish study concluded that fish consumption could be associated with decreased risk of prostate cancer. P. Terry, P. Lichtenstein,

M. Feychting et al., Fatty fish consumption and risk of prostate cancer, *Lancet* 357 (2001): 1764–1766.

18 K. Augustsson, D. S. Michaud, E. B. Rimm et al., A prospective study of intake of fish and marine fatty acids and prostate cancer, *Cancer Epidemiology, Biomarkers and Prevention* 12 (2003): 64–67.

19 P. Terry, A. Wolk, H. Vainio et al., Fatty fish consumption lowers the risk of endometrial cancer: A nationwide case-control study in Sweden, *Cancer Epidemiology, Biomarkers and Prevention* 11 (2002): 143–145.

20 R. A. Murphy, M. S. Wilke, M. Perrine et al., Loss of adipose tissue and plasma phospholipids: Relationship to survival in advanced cancer patients, *Clinical Nutrition* 29 (2010): 482–487.

21 Dr. William Harris, Personal communication, December 2010.

22 I. Newton, Companion animal omega-3's: Market size, trends, and product concepts with fish oil, presentation at Conference on Omega-3s for Cosmetics, Pet Foods, Dietary Supplements, August 2011, www.smarts hortcourses.com.

23 For a detailed explanation of the FDA recommendation, see Food and Drug Administration, Letter responding to health claim petition: Omega-3 fatty acids and reduced risk of coronary heart disease, September 8, 2004, www.fda.gov/Food/LabelingNutrition/LabelClaims/ QualifiedHealthClaims/ucm072936.htm.

Chapter 12 Selecting and Preparing Safe Seafood

1. E. N. Ponnampalam, N. J. Mann, and A. J. Sinclair, Effect of feeding systems on omega-3 fatty acids, conjugated linoleic acid and trans fatty acids in Australian beef cuts: Potential impact on human health, *Asia Pacific Journal of Clinical Nutrition* 15 (2006): 21–29.

2. Z. Lu, T. C. Chen, A. Zhang et al., An evaluation of the vitamin D3 content in fish: Is the vitamin D content adequate to satisfy the dietary requirement for vitamin D? *Journal of Steroid Biochemistry and Molecular Biology* 103 (2007): 642–644.

3. Y. Nagaki, M. Mihara, J. Takahashi et al., The effect of astaxanthin on retinal capillary blood flow in normal volunteers, *Journal of Clinical Therapeutics and Medicines* 21 (2005): 537–542.

4. B. Capelli with G. Cysewski, *Natural Astaxanthin: King of the Carotenoids* (Cyanotech Corp., 2007); F. J. Pashkow, D. G. Watumull, and C. L. Campbell, Astaxanthin: A novel potential treatment for oxidative stress and inflammation in cardiovascular disease, *American Jour-*

nal of Cardiology 101: 58D–68D; J. S. Park, J. H. Chyun, Y. K. Kim et al., Astaxanthin decreased oxidative stress and inflammation and enhanced immune response in humans, *Nutrition and Metabolism* 7 (2010): 18; G. Richardson, How astaxanthin combats degenerative disease, *Life Extension Magazine*, July 2011.

5. An analysis of data from eleven thousand British women found no evidence that consumption of more than three portions of seafood a week during pregnancy has an adverse effect on the child. In contrast, maternal consumption of more than 340 grams (12 ounces) of seafood per week was beneficial for the child's neurodevelopment. This is the study that supports the recommendation to eat 12 ounces of seafood per week. J. R. Hibbeln, J. M. Davis, C. Steer et al., Maternal seafood consumption in pregnancy and neurodevelopmental outcomes in childhood (ALSPAC study), *Lancet* 369 (2007): 578–585.

This is an excellent review article giving scientific evidence that the health benefits of seafood far outweigh the possible risks. D. Mozaffarian and E. B. Rimm, Fish intake, contaminants, and human health: Evaluating the risks and the benefits, *JAMA* 296 (2006): 1885–1899. Another excellent review is: J. T. Brenna and A. Lapillonne, Background paper on fat and fatty acid requirements during pregnancy and lactation, *Nutrition and Metabolism* 55 (2009): 97–122.

6. These authors studied selenium-mercury interactions and concluded that people who eat selenium-rich fish suffer no health effects from mercury. L. Raymond and N. V. Ralston, Mercury: Selenium interactions and health implications, *Seychelles Medical and Dental Journal* 7 (Nov. 2004): 72–77. See also J. J. Kaneko and N. V. Ralston, Selenium and mercury in pelagic fish in the central north Pacific near Hawaii, *Biological Trace Element Research* 119 (2007): 242–254.

7. MSC's website is at www.msc.org. For more about Alaskan fisheries, see Commercial fisheries: Information by fishery, Alaska Department of Fish and Game, www.adfg.alaska.gov.

8. J. R. Hibbeln, L. Nieminen, T. L. Blasbalg et al., Healthy intakes of n-3 and n-6 fatty acids: Estimations considering worldwide diversity, *American Journal of Clinical Nutrition* 83 (2006): S1483–S1493.

Index

. . .

About the Authors

• • •

William Sears, MD, is the author of more than thirty bestselling books on parenting and the pediatric expert on whom American parents increasingly rely for advice and information on all aspects of pregnancy, birth, childcare, and family nutrition. Dr. Sears received his pediatric training at Harvard Medical School's Children's Hospital and Toronto's Hospital for Sick Children. He has practiced pediatrics for more than forty years and is an associate clinical professor at the University of California, Irvine, School of Medicine. He is the father of eight children and lives with his wife, Martha, in southern California.

James Sears, MD, FAAP, is a board-certified pediatrician in practice with his father and brother. He has two children and has authored six books on parenting and nutrition. Dr. Sears gives daily medical advice to millions as the cohost of the Emmy Award–winning talk show *The Doctors,* which is syndicated in twenty-two countries around the world. He frequently travels the country speaking about the vital role omega-3 nutrition plays in a variety of medical and behavioral problems.